D0753197

X

EMERGENCY!

The Active Horseman's Book of Emergency Care

KAREN E.N. HAYES, DVM, MS

Half Halt Press, Inc.
Boonsboro, Maryland

Emergency!
The Active Horseman's Book of Emergency Care
© 1995 Karen E.N. Hayes, DVM, MS

Published in the United States of America by
Half Halt Press, Inc.
P.O. Box 67
Boonsboro, MD 21713

Text illustrations © 1995 Karen E.N. Hayes, DVM, MS
Photographs by the author

Jacket and cover design by Gallagher Wood Design

Emergency! The Active Horseman's Book of Emergency Care is not intended as a substitute or replacement for appropriate veterinary care. The author and publisher strongly encourage all horse owners to seek out the best medical advice and care available from a licensed veterinarian.

Library of Congress Cataloging-in-Publication Data

Hayes, Karen E.N.
    Emergency! : the active horseman's book of emergency care / Karen
E.N. Hayes
        p.   cm.
    Includes index.
    ISBN 0-939481-42-1
    1. Horses--Wounds and injuries--Treatment.   2. Horses--Diseases--
Treatment 3. Veterinary emergencies. 4. First aid for animals.
I. Title.
SF951.H325 1995   95-20091
636.1'0896025--dc20   CIP

Table of Contents

Introduction

I
t's every horse owner's worst nightmare: you and your horse are out there somewhere — on the trail, or at a remote mountain campsite, or on the way to or from an equine event — out there in the middle of some veterinary no-man's land — and your horse is hurt or sick. You'd summon a vet, *any* vet, if you could. But you can't — you're going to have to hunt one down first. For the moment you're on your own, and your horse is counting on you.

If you haven't been in a situation like this yet, rest assured that if you own horses long enough, you'll come to accept emergency equine care as something that goes with the territory. And although the ideal would be to have a veterinarian on the scene immediately, the unfortunate truth is, very few emergency situations are... well, *ideal*. In fifteen years as a veterinarian, I've seen too many simple, completely resolvable emergency situations turn fatal because veterinary care couldn't be provided fast enough and the horse owner had no idea how to exercise a little damage control.

And then there's the other problem — the problem of all the free advice that's floating out there in the horse world. Like the old cowboy's colic remedy: hold a saucer of turpentine against the horse's navel, and he'll magically "suck it up" and suddenly feel fine. The turpentine "treatment" has also been advocated as a remedy for founder. There are enough bad recommendations out there to fill a book of their own, and unfortunately not all of those recommendations are so obviously ridiculous — some of them sound just sensible enough to induce a desperate horse owner to give them a try, and the horse's well being hangs in the balance. What makes it all the more dangerous from the horse's point of view is the fact that most horse owners have some veterinary drugs in their tack room — medications they picked up at a feed store, or bought through a mail order catalog, or obtained from a veterinarian — and they've had no guidance in their proper use. When faced with a crisis, they're apt to do the human thing: *do something,* even if it turns out to be the wrong thing.

This book is designed to give you a clear picture of what's going on inside when your horse is in the middle of a medical crisis. Then it'll walk you through some logical, practical, and powerful treatments that can improve his chances of getting through his crisis with life and limb intact. If you understand what's happening to your horse, you'll understand the logic behind the right treatment, and you'll see why some treatments will not only fail to help but will actually make the situation worse. You'll learn how to assess your situation, to decide what can and can't wait, and to take steps to improve the odds that when you find a competent equine veterinarian to take over for you, you can hand him/her a lead rope attached to a horse with the best possible chance of recovering from this crisis, preferably unscathed, and returning to full performance as quickly as possible.

Drugs, the Law, the Insurance Company, & Event Regulations

I t's against the law to practice veterinary medicine without a valid veterinary license. What this means is that any time you administer any kind of treatment — not just prescription drugs, but *any* treatment, including bandages — to someone else's horse, you could be breaking the law. The law was written by lawmakers, not veterinarians, and when it's enforced, it's enforced by the same officials that collar hard-boiled criminals.

Taking care of your own animals is another matter. Fact is, if you stood by and allowed your horse to suffer, you might have another group of lawmakers on your back. More to the point, you'd have trouble sleeping at night.

Know the law. Use this book to help you care for your own horse, to bridge the disastrous gap that often exists between your discovery of a serious health problem and your ability to find, and procure, competent equine veterinary assistance.

Drugs and the law

There are a lot of different laws and a lot of different agencies in the federal and state governments that have a say-so in the matter of who can and who can't possess and administer certain drugs to animals. If you're not extremely careful, you can step on the toes of the USDA (United States Department of Agriculture), the FDA CVM (Food and Drug Administration Center for Veterinary Medicine), the EPA (Environmental Protection Agency), the DEA (Drug Enforcement Agency), and the vagaries of 50 different state governments, and you and your source for the drugs you carry for your horse could end up behind bars with a stiff (up to $250,000) fine.

What makes this a complex issue is that, despite laws that are quite strict in their wording and intent, for decades it's been no big deal for the average Joe to walk into a country feed store, or call the 800 number of some veterinary supply catalog, and simply select and pay for just about anything he needs to care for his animals, from vaccines to antibiotics to antiinflammatories to tranquilizers. Tell the buyers and the suppliers that it's illegal and you're likely to get a reaction of disbelief, resentment and scorn. They don't believe you, and if you want to make a stink about it, they'll just do their business with someone else.

Well, whether they like it or not, the laws are explicit, and for a number of reasons those laws are beginning to get renewed attention within the federal and state governments. The control of the possession and sale of veterinary drugs has become a high-priority issue.

Why all the fuss? Veterinarians, livestock producers, animal trainers, and feed store owners have been buying and selling prescription drugs for years and years, often using them in ways for which they were never intended, while the laws gathered dust and were largely ignored. Why the sudden hardball attitude on the part of government? Does anybody really believe that you're going to shoot yourself up with Banamine™, or sell a syringeful of acepromazine to a neighborhood kid?

No, it's nothing like that. Most of the fracas got started because of the hard-working, independent, self-sufficient livestock producer who operates on a very narrow profit margin and thinks he can't afford to call the vet every time a calf gets the snots. So he stocks up on all the drugs he's seen the vet use over the years and administers them himself to save on big vet bills. Fact is, he may make some catastrophic errors from time to time, but overall he does pretty well for himself. Sure, he's indirectly insulting the vet by implying that all there is to practicing veterinary medicine is filling a syringe with penicillin, ramming the needle through the animal's thick hide, and pumping the stuff in. But insulting vets is not what this is all about. It's about your health and mine.

Here's the real issue. There are a lot of people with drug allergies, drug sensitivities, or a tendency for adverse side-effects from many different kinds of drugs. Many of those drugs are or were used routinely in the care of milk- or meat-producing animals, from chickens to catfish to beef and dairy cows to hogs. Young meat-producing animals grow faster when antibiotics are mixed into their feed and given daily, even when they aren't sick. Implants are inserted under their skin to release hormones for the same reason — bigger, faster growth with no increase in feed. Hormones can make dairy cows give more milk, and they can make baby chicks grow into fat, meaty fryers in six short weeks. You can't blame the farmer for thinking this is a good thing — it's like getting something for nothing. And even if he's uncomfortable with it, his neighbor is doing it and getting bigger dividends at the livestock sales, so he feels forced to participate in order to compete.

Trouble is, tiny residues of drugs in the meat or milk of these animals can end up on your dinner table, and if you happen to be one of those people who will die if exposed to chloramphenicol, or if you're allergic to penicillin, or if you just aren't too keen on the idea of having your milk or steak laced with steroids and sex hormones, well, it's for your sake that those laws were written. It's an issue that really does warrant government focus, as evidenced by the Puerto Rican outbreak of hormonal imbalances in children a decade ago — little girls as young as 5 and 6 were developing breasts, thanks to estrogen (the female hormone) in dairy milk. Dairymen had been administering the hormone to their cows to boost feed efficiency and milk production.

And so the old, forgotten laws have been dusted off and resurrected, and government agencies are cracking down in a very big way. But, you say, with all due respect for the laws, my horse isn't being raised for the meat market. So can I have "bute" and Banamine™ and a few of the tranquilizers and antibiotics to use on my horse?

Can you have prescription items on hand for emergency use in your horse?

Well, you're free to purchase and use all the over-the-counter (OTC) medications you want for your horse — there's no law against that, and there is an impressive array of very effective products available this way, with no prescription, no hassle. And prescription items get "downgraded" to OTC status from time to time when officials decide that they've been around long enough for people to become familiar with their proper use — this has recently happened with some of the human-use drugs like ibuprofen, imodium, some antihistamines, and medications for vaginal yeast infections. Is that because somebody decided they're not dangerous any more? No, it's because the decision makers decided that average, non-medical personnel have had enough experience with these medications now that they can be trusted to buy and use them safely, without a physician's guidance. The same is true of many veterinary drugs, including dewormers, some vaccines, and some antibiotics (including penicillin, tetracycline, and, recently, gentamicin).

But drugs that remain in the "prescription" category are still restricted because there are too many complexities or hazards associated with their improper use, and the regulatory agencies worry that people won't use them safely unless they first get one-on-one instructions from a veterinarian.

One of those potential hazards is overdose: with some drugs, figuring proper dose depends not only on knowing the animal's approximate weight and being able to do some simple math, but also on knowing what conditions might make the potential side-effects of that medication unacceptably risky, in which case the usual dose should be dramatically reduced. Xylazine (Rompun™), for example, is a wonderful sedative in horses that even has some pain-killing properties — it's invaluable in facilitating the treatment of a number of very common ailments and injuries in horses. But one of its side-effects is respiratory depression, and if a well-meaning but ignorant owner gives just a little too much to a young foal, or to an aged horse, or to any horse with a respiratory problem (and that problem might not be obvious), that ordinarily insignificant side-effect becomes very significant, possibly life-threatening. Give a sedative to any horse that's overly excited, and you could actually cause his blood pressure to drop too low too fast, and he'll faint. Maybe even fall on top of you. And even when a horse is heavily sedated with xylazine or its newer cousin, detomidine, he still retains the ability to deliver a well-aimed kick. Lawmakers know that these "details" about drugs aren't readily available to the average horse owner, and so they leave the more complicated drugs in the "prescription only" category.

Here's another hazard associated with xylazine: the proper dose for a cow is about 1/100 of the proper dose for a horse of the same weight. Most people don't know that. If you've used xylazine before on your horses, you might think you're pretty familiar with it. So you might figure it'd be great for sedating your nasty cow so you can treat her foot rot without getting your head kicked off, and you calculate the dose based on what a *horse* of her weight would require. If you're not educated in veterinary pharmacology, you're going to kill the cow with the sedative — your seemingly conservative 2-cc dose will overdose her by 100 times, and she'll simply slip into a deep sleep and never wake up. You know as well as I do that people do things like this all the time. It's one of the reasons for the law.

But, you say, if I want to kill my own cow because of my own stupidity, that's my business. I suppose that's true, but there's another issue that must be addressed: When a drug is in the "prescription drug" category, whenever possible it is dispensed in child-proof containers. Even if you might argue that some hapless cow's life isn't important, the drug control agencies take a very serious stance on the life of a curious child whose mother is busy mucking out stalls and hasn't noticed that the kid is playing with the medicine box in the tack room.

You're absolutely right if you think that the jar of pine tar, and the bottle of aspirin, and the jug of antifreeze, and the bucket of mineral supplements pose more of a danger to an unsupervised child than a bottle of Banamine™ that really isn't a threat until somebody pulls a dose of the stuff into an armed syringe. In fact, as far as the child's safety is concerned, the horse itself is a heck of a lot more dangerous than that bottle of Banamine™. In that regard, and since Banamine™ has been in use for over a decade, I wouldn't be at all surprised if sometime in the near future it joins the ranks of familiar over-the-counter veterinary drugs. It seems that just about every active performance horse person has a bottle of it and uses it on his or her horse, despite the law. But until the law changes, the fact remains that, legally, you should not have Banamine™, or any other prescription drug, in your possession unless you have a prescription for it, no matter how easy it is for you to get that drug without a prescription.

This shifts the attention to the person giving the prescription: the veterinarian. A veterinarian who dispenses prescription drugs to a person he/she doesn't even know for an animal he/she has never seen is breaking the law and not only risks losing his/her license to practice veterinary medicine but could actually end up with that aforementioned stiff fine and real jail time. How do you know if it's a prescription drug when you see it?

- It's a prescription drug if the label reads,

  "Caution: Federal law restricts this drug to use by or on the order of a licensed veterinarian"

- But it's an over-the counter drug if the label reads,

  "for veterinary use only,"
  "sold only to licensed veterinarians,"

or if it bears no reference to veterinarians at all.

Confused? I don't blame you. To make it even more confusing, some drugs are labelled as prescription under one brand name and OTC under another, depending on what type of animal the label says they're for.

The prescription drugs

In order for a prescription to be considered legitimate in the eyes of the law, there must be what the law calls a veterinarian-client-patient relationship: the vet must have spoken to the client about the proper use of the drug and its potential hazards, have reasonable expectations that the client can and will follow those instructions, and the prescription must be intended for a specific animal or herd of animals with which the veterinarian is familiar and upon which the veterinarian has laid his/her actual hands in the recent past.

For the protection of humans that might come into contact with the drug accidentally, the prescription drug must bear a label with information needed by emergency room personnel. The label must identify the name, amount and strength of the active ingredients, the proper dose for the intended animal, how it should be given, the date of the prescription, the name, address, and telephone number of the prescriber, the name of the animal it's intended for, and the name of the animal's owner. If you walk into a vet's office and demand that he/she sell you a prescription item with no questions asked, you're asking him/her to break the law and jeopardize his/her business, livelihood, and personal life. No matter how valuable a customer you might be, it's doubtful that your patronage is worth that risk.

But what about the highly experienced horse person, who owns and performs with a valuable horse, who has a very close working relationship with his/her regular veterinarian, who is well acquainted with the techniques used for examining and medicating horses, and who simply wants to have on hand a limited supply of a few often-used prescription drugs — just in case the horse falls victim to one of several injuries or ailments that commonly afflict horses during the rigors and stresses of travel and performance? In my opinion, it's a reasonable request, but ultimately it's up to *your* veterinarian. If you are an intelligent, responsible, experienced horse person, and your veterinarian knows you well enough to know that you can be trusted to

1. recognize the common emergency conditions outlined in this book,

2. follow recommended guidelines for the emergency use of the drugs discussed in this book,

3. contact the home veterinary office to report what has happened and receive further instructions, and

4. move heaven and earth to get your horse to the nearest competent equine veterinarian for immediate follow-up and continued care if the horse can't wait for you to get him all the way home,

then your veterinarian might decide, at his/her discretion, to dispense a prescription drug for your use on that specific animal under those specific circumstances, should they ever occur. To legitimize this decision, your vet should be sure to apply the aforementioned label. Physicians do this sort of thing all the time — it's not unusual for a family doctor to write a prescription for antibiotics and a strong pain killer for you to take on a backpacking trip *just in case* you should happen to break a leg while you're out in the middle of nowhere. Your doctor knows if he can trust you and he acts accordingly.

If, on the other hand, a veterinarian hardly knows you, or is unfamiliar with your horse, or has any reason to suspect that you might misjudge or abuse or misuse the privelege of possessing any prescription drugs as a safeguard against future mishaps, then that veterinarian is well advised to refuse your request. Again, keeping you happy might be important to your veterinarian, but not important enough to risk losing a veterinary license and gaining a federal conviction. If your veterinarian isn't comfortable that you have a legitimate veterinarian-client-patient relationship and that you are capable of acting as his/her agent in an emergency situation, he/she *shouldn't* give you that prescription.

With all of the above in mind, the latest recommendations on the use of prescription items that you might have in your possession to help your horse in the face of a crisis will be explained in the appropriate chapters of this book. The purpose for discussing the proper use of these prescription drugs is not to advocate or encourage their use, but rather to prevent their improper use — to help ensure that you will not harm your horse simply because you meant well, were in a panic, and got your hands on the drugs without guidance. If your veterinarian agrees to dispense these prescription items to you for emergency use, the recommendations in this book will accompany the specific instructions you receive from your veterinarian when you obtain the prescription. If your veterinarian's instructions conflict with the recommendations in this book, you should follow your vet's instructions by default, since he/she knows your animal.

If your veterinarian refuses to prescribe emergency medications for possible future crises, accept his/her judgement. You can still deal with your crisis according to the non-prescription recommendations in this book — in other words, even if you don't have those prescription items, there are still plenty of powerful and effective OTC medications available, plenty of things you can do to help your horse while you're working to locate veterinary assistance.

Performance Event Regulations

As far as event regulations are concerned, the safest thing for you to do if your horse becomes ill or injured and requires medical treatment when you're on the way to an event is to concentrate on dealing with the crisis and withdraw from the event. However, some crises are very short-lived and quickly resolved with prompt, proper treatment, and you might want to go ahead with your plans to compete in the event after all. But what about the drugs that are now circulating in your horse's system? Will he be disqualified?

That depends on many things. Small, local horse events often have no rules about drug use and don't do any drug testing, but most of the larger equine events — state fairs, shows, endurance races, etc., abide by the drug rules and regulations set forth by the American Horse Shows Association (AHSA) and the Federation Equestre Internationale (FEI). Events under their jurisdiction will adhere to the strict letter of AHSA and/or FEI law. It's your responsibility to find out whether or not your event follows a particular set of rules regarding drugs — you're much better off withdrawing your horse ahead of time than finding out later that he is in violation of the event's regulations and has been disqualified. Such disqualification could not only cost you a victory at the event, it could permanently tarnish your reputation and suspend you from future events.

Rules and Regulations of the AHSA

The fee collected from each entrant into an AHSA event pays for blood or urine drug testing of the participants. The drug tests look for three different types of substances:

1. any detectable amount of drugs that might affect a horse's performance (*see table 1*),

---

THE AGENCIES ARE WATCHING YOU

☞ The Food and Drug Administration Center for Veterinary Medicine: regulates veterinary drugs, animal feeds, and medicated feeds

☞ The United States Department of Agriculture: regulates vaccines and antitoxins

☞ The Environmental Protection Agency: regulates insecticides, disinfectants, and rodenticides

☞ The Drug Enforcement Agency: regulates substances with a high potential for abuse or addiction

2. too much of a drug that is allowed only at specified low levels (see *Table 3),* and

3. any detectable amount of drugs that might "trick" the drug test into missing the presence of forbidden drugs (see *Table 2).*

Note that the lists are not complete — a complete list of all forbidden drugs would be as big as the New York phone book — so only those drugs that might be used legitimately to deal with a problem in your particular horse are listed. In other words, it's assumed that your motivation for giving a drug is not to "cheat" in performance, but rather to treat an abnormality. If that assumption is not misplaced, the tables should be helpful.

Phenylbutazone, flunixin meglumine (Banamine™), & ketoprofen (Ketofen™)

These three antiiflammatory drugs are used so commonly to deal with the aches and pains of performance horses that the AHSA has given them special consideration. Although their recommendations do not guarantee that your horse will not be disqualified, AHSA officials have gone to a great deal of trouble to investigate some of the characteristics of bute and Banamine™ and Ketofen™ in the horse's system so that you can better judge whether or not your horse will be eligible to compete. For a summary of their recommendations, see *Table 4.*

Methocarbamol (Robaxin-V™)

The muscle relaxant methocarbamol (Robaxin-V™) is most often used in horses with a history of tying-up (myositis). It can only be given in tablet form to competing horses, because the injectable form contains polyethylene glycol, which is a forbidden masking substance. If the injectable is used, you have to file a medication document with the steward/technical delegate as described below (page 12), and follow the associated regulations as detailed. When tablets are used, the dose should be accurately calculated and not more than 500 mg/100 lb bodyweight should be given per 12-hour period. This means a maximum dose of 5 grams (ten 500-mg tablets) every 12 hours for a 1000 lb horse. No dose can be given during the 6-hour period prior to the competition.

TABLE 1

DRUGS THAT MAY AFFECT PERFORMANCE
THAT ARE FORBIDDEN BY AHSA RULES

D=depressant   S=stimulant   LA=local anesthetic

Acepromazine (a common tranquilizer): D

Aminophylline (prescribed for horses with heaves): S

Chlorpheniramine (an antihistamine prescribed for horses with signs of allergy): S

Clenbuterol (a bronchodilator for horses with heaves and other respiratory ailments): S

Detomidine (a sedative & painkiller for minor surgical procedures in the awake horse): D

Dextromethorphan (a cough suppressant): D

Diazepam (aka Valium™, a sedative and anti-seizure medication): D

Diphenhydramine (an antihistamine prescribed for horses with signs of allergy): S

Guaifenesin (an expectorant): D

Lidocaine (a local anesthetic and a heart medication): LA

Mepivicaine (a relatively long-acting [4 hrs ±] local anesthetic used for nerve blocks): LA

Morphine (a sedative for standing minor surgery and a cough suppressant): S

Pentazocine (aka Talwin™, a sedative and a pain killer): S

Phenobarbital (a sedative and an anti-seizure medication): D

Phenytoin (aka Dilantin™, an anti-seizure medication): D

Procaine (an additive in the white, creamy penicillin injectable products): LA

Promazine (a tranquilizer from the same family of drugs as acepromazine): D

Theophylline (a bronchodilator for horses with heaves and other respiratory ailments): S

Tripelennamine (an antihistamine for horses with signs of allergy): S

Xylazine (aka Rompun™, a sedative and painkiller): D

TABLE 2

EXAMPLES OF DRUGS THAT MAY MASK
THE PRESENCE OF AHSA-FORBIDDEN DRUGS

Benzimidazole anthelmintics (Telmin™, Omnizole™, TBZ™, Panacur™, Benzelmin™)

Dipyrone (aka Novin™, a mild pain killer and antispasmodic for spasmodic colic)

Furosemide (aka Lasix™, a diuretic)

Isoxsuprine (a vasodilator sometimes used in acute laminitis)

Polyethylene Glycol (a preservative found in many injectable medications)

Sulfa (an antimicrobial product commonly combined with trimethoprim)

Trimethoprim (an antimicrobial product commonly combined with a sulfa)

TABLE 3

EXAMPLES OF RESTRICTED DRUGS

(LEVELS ABOVE PRE-SET AMOUNTS ARE FORBIDDEN)

Phenylbutazone (antiinflammatory and pain killer)
Flunixin (Banamine™) (antiinflammatory, pain killer, and anti-endotoxin)
Methocarbamol (Robaxin-V™) (a muscle relaxant)

So, is your horse disqualified if you (or a veterinarian) administered medications prior to the competition? When in doubt, the answer is probably yes — he's disqualified. Following are the specific circumstances under which he *might* still be eligible to participate in the event:

1. There's a legitimate, *medical* reason for having given the medication (not just that it made him easier to handle or load into the trailer, for example),

2. At least 24 hours will lapse between the time the medication was given and the time the horse is to perform,

3. It was given by a licensed veterinarian or, if the vet was not available, by the trainer (which could be you),

4. You've documented, in writing, the identification of the horse, the name of the drug, the dose, time and mode of administration, and the reason it was considered necessary,

5. You've given this documentation to the steward or technical official at the competition within one hour of having given the treatment to the horse, or within one hour that the official reported to duty, or within one hour that the horse arrived on the grounds, whichever applies to your situation, and

6. That official has signed your document and written in the date and time he/she signed it.

If you and your horse meet all six of the above requirements, you *might* be able to comply with the event's regulations and compete legally. However, you might still be in trouble. Some drugs take a *long* time to be cleared from the blood or urine of your horse, possibly showing up on drug tests done as many as 72 hours after the drug was given. Even if you follow all the rules of documentation and so forth, you'll still be disqualified if your horse fails the drug test. Every horse is different, and a drug that might be cleared from one horse's system within 12 hours might still be lingering in another horse's system several hours later. Don't stake your reputation on the hope that your horse's metabolism is "average."

Non-medical drug use

If you use any drug on a horse for any reason other than medical (for example, if you give a drug to calm him down so you can clip him, or load him in the trailer), this is considered a forbidden drugging and you must keep the horse out of competition until all traces of that drug have disappeared from his system and will not show up at all on blood or urine drug tests. Rule of thumb: a minimum of seven days' withdrawal for any forbidden substance, and 14 days if it contains any local anesthetic. And you might need more than 30 days if you use any slow-release, long-acting substances or if you give more than one dose of any drug.

TABLE 4

AHSA RECOMMENDATIONS FOR PHENYLBUTAZONE, FLUNIXIN MEGLUMINE (BANAMINE™) AND KETOPROFEN (KETOFEN™)

1. If your horse needs phenylbutazone or flunixin meglumine or ketoprofen, no more than one of those three should be used. If two are given within 7 days of the event, neither should have been given within 48 hours of the event or the likelihood of failing the drug test will be high.

2. When phenylbutazone is given the dose should be accurately calculated, should never exceed the maximal dose of 0.2 g/100 lb every 24 hours, and it should not be given for more than 4 days in a row. No maximal dose should be given within 24 hours prior to the event, and none should be given within 12 hours prior to the event.

3. When flunixin meglumine is given the dose should be accurately calculated, should never exceed the maximal dose of 50 mg/100 lb body weight every 24 hours, and it should not be given for more than 4 days in a row. No maximal dose should be given within 24 hours prior to the event, and none should be given within 12 hours prior to the event.

4. When ketoprofen is given the dose should be accurately calculated and should never exceed the maximal dose of 0.1 g/100 lb body weight every 24 hours. No repeat doses should be given sooner than 24 hours after the previous dose, and it should not be given for more than 4 days in a row. None should be given within 12 hours prior to the event.

The bottom line: if you're a performance horse person, it pays to be very, *very* choosy about the use of drugs in your performance horse.

Culpability

No matter who gave the drug to the horse, it's the trainer that the AHSA considers to be responsible for making sure the horse complies with the rules and regulations, and therefore it is upon the trainer's neck that the axe will fall if the horse comes up "dirty" on a drug test. Violations are published in the NOTICE OF PENALTY section of Horse Show Magazine and can ruin a trainer's career.

Rules and Regulations of the FEI

FEI-sanctioned events, which include Olympic equestrian sports, are even more strict than the AHSA events regarding drugs: any traces of any drugs or medications are forbidden. You must, therefore, be extremely careful to observe the withdrawal times for any drugs that your horse might receive at any time prior to an FEI-sanctioned event, and you must remember that every horse is an individual, and your horse might require longer to eliminate a particular drug from his system than would the average horse. Don't take chances with your horse performance career: when in doubt, withdraw from competition. If your horse turns up drug-positive on a test, you will receive no extra consideration for his failure to follow the rule of thumb about a 7-day withdrawal for most forbidden substances.

Under FEI regulations, if some sort of treatment is required, and your horse has already been entered into some future event, you must get advance approval from the event's veterinary officials to give that treatment if you still intend to compete, you must report the treatment in writing to the event's officials, and you must receive permission and approval of the ground jury before participating in competition after that treatment.

Will my insurance company honor my policy if I do my own emergency treatment?

Every insurance company has its own set of rules, laid down by the underwriters' organizations that provide the financial backing for the companies. Technically, according to the legalese that forms the "magna carta" of a livestock insurance company, insurance companies are well within their legal rights to deny a claim for treatment costs and/or losses when any portion of the care was provided by someone other than a licensed veterinarian. According to the letter of that legal wording, "care" means the administration of anything other than unadulterated food and water. We're right back to that original statement at the beginning of this chapter — that it's illegal to apply a leg wrap ("practice veterinary medicine") without a license. It may seem preposterous, you may not like it, but it's legal. If you're smart, you'll bend over backward to comply with it.

But there's good news. Most of the reputable livestock insurance companies, and specifically those that insure a lot of horses, are flexible and reasonable people. If they're "horsey" themselves, the claims adjusters understand only too well how things can go wrong with horses, and how difficult it can be to find professional help when you're in unfamiliar territory. Even representatives of the "main" equine veterinary association have stated that over the next decade or so it will become more and more difficult to find a good equine vet, thanks to rising practice standards, rising business and equipment costs, the slumping horse industry, and the clustering of good practitioners in a few, high-density horse communities like Lexington, Ocala, upstate New York, and so forth. I spoke with some of those reasonable, horsey claims adjusters, and here's the consensus:

First of all, choose your insurer carefully. Talk not only to the people who enroll new accounts, but also to the people who handle the claims. Find out if they're experienced horse people, and how long they've been with the company. Ask them, point blank, what they would want you to do if you were in a crisis with your horse and there was no veterinarian available to help — would they frown on first-aid treatment administered by you or your trainer, even if you've been instructed in advance by your veterinarian?

Once you've chosen your insurer, be sure to mention at the outset that you intend, if circumstances dictate, to take steps to help your horse in a crisis. Get a note from your veterinarian, stating that he/she vouches for your ability as an educated, level-headed, equine-experienced person who can be trusted to do what's necessary in an emergency, but that you're not a "do-it-yourselfer" by nature — in other words, you have a good working relationship with your veterinarian and are, therefore, a responsible horseperson. Submit this note along with your application and insist that it be in your file in case of a claim. Keep a copy for yourself. Understand that this doesn't guarantee you anything — a claim could still be denied — but in my experience, adjusters with the well-established companies are very accommodating and understanding.

If it's absolutely mandatory that there never be any question about any potential claims, you're probably already breaking the rules (Do you give your own vaccines? Spray wound medication on scrapes? Give medicated shampoos?) and you'll want to become informed before you continue.

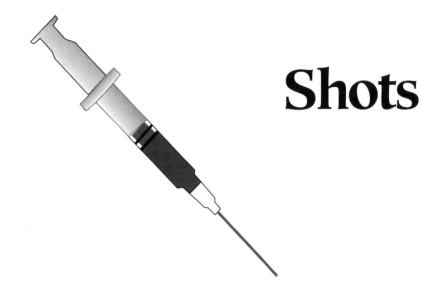

Shots

Hopefully your veterinarian has already taught you the proper technique for administering intramuscular injections to your horse. The location you choose is generally a matter of personal preference — yours and your horse's. Some horses object strenuously to "butt shots" but stand like angels for an injection in the side of the neck. Some owners are queasy about certain locations and more at ease with others. It really doesn't matter, as long as you do it right.

There are two hazards to avoid:

1. accidental injection into a blood vessel, and
2. infection.

Follow these simple steps and you should be able to avoid these hazards every time.

Choose your injection site

Choose one of the 4 locations indicated, paying close attention to anatomic details that must be avoided. In the neck, the vertebrae and the spinal cord they protect are arranged in a backward S-shape from poll to chest. Outline this with your hand before selecting your injection site. The broad elastic band (the *ligamentum nuchae)* along the crest of the neck is often victimized by inexperienced injectors — stay away from it too. In the croup, stay in the middle of the thick muscle "hammock" that is slung from the points of the bony pelvis and the sacrum. To avoid "pooling" of the medication, which can irritate the tissues and cause an abscess, stay away from horizontal muscles — instead, choose a spot where there's a slope, to aid in dispersal of the medication (see illustration). In the upper rear leg, the sciatic nerve must be avoided by grasping the straplike muscles at the back of the thigh to push the nerve forward, then inserting the needle into that handful of muscle while aiming it backwards, away from the nerve. The brisket area at the front of the breast is prone to "pooling" of injectable substances, which can lead to abscess formation, because of gravity and the looseness of the tissues there — deep injection usually avoids this problem, but it's probably best to stay away from this site unless you have no choice.

Clean the site

Swabbing the injection site with rubbing alcohol does not, alas, sterilize it. But it can help to clean off dust, since the dust will adhere to a moist cloth. A logical alternative is to choose a site that's relatively clean to begin with, curry and dust-brush it to remove lingering dust and dander, then wipe it to a gloss with a soft, clean, slightly damp cloth. You can use rubbing alcohol if it makes you feel better, but unless you allow the tissues to soak in it for 30 minutes, it's probably no more effective than clear water. Always clean off the top of the bottle's stopper before inserting the needle, always use a brand new, sterile, disposable hypodermic needle and syringe, and use a second needle to inject the horse (not, in other words, the same needle you used to draw up the medication from the bottle). This two-needle policy serves three purposes: it avoids pricking the horse's skin with any germs that might be living on the stopper, it ensures that the horse's skin will be pierced with a perfectly sharp needle, and it avoids introducing any of the medication until the tip of the needle is where you intend for it to be.

Insert the needle separately

For an adult horse, use an 18- or 19-gauge, 1-1/2" needle. Detach it from the syringe and insert it, in one smooth motion, all the way up to its hub. Lean over and look into the hub for any backflow of blood. None? Good, you can continue. (But if there *is* any hint of blood in there, pull the needle out and start over with a fresh

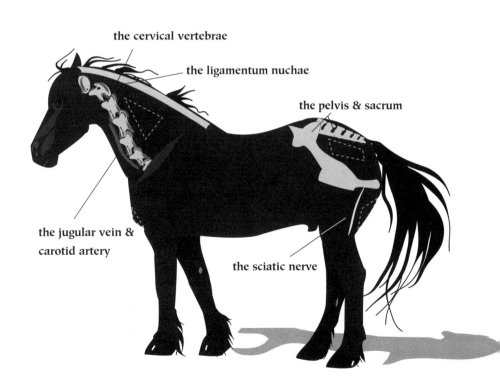

the cervical vertebrae

the ligamentum nuchae

the pelvis & sacrum

the jugular vein & carotid artery

the sciatic nerve

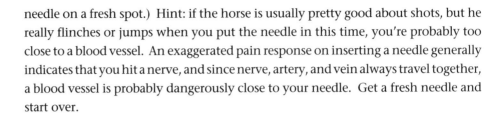

needle on a fresh spot.) Hint: if the horse is usually pretty good about shots, but he really flinches or jumps when you put the needle in this time, you're probably too close to a blood vessel. An exaggerated pain response on inserting a needle generally indicates that you hit a nerve, and since nerve, artery, and vein always travel together, a blood vessel is probably dangerously close to your needle. Get a fresh needle and start over.

Attach the syringe and pull back the plunger

While one hand rests against the horse and steadies the hub of the needle, attach the syringe with the other hand. Now pull back slightly on the plunger of the syringe and watch to see if you've pulled any blood up into the medication. No? Good, you can continue. (But if there's even a *wisp* of blood pulled back into the syringe, you've entered a blood vessel — maybe just a tiny one. Pull out and start over with fresh supplies and a fresh spot.)

Inject the medication

Slowly inject the medication by pushing on the plunger with one hand while holding the hub of the needle steady with the other. Figure on injecting one cc of substance in about five seconds' time. Stop midway through the injection and pull back on the plunger once more, just to be sure the needle hasn't moved and pierced a blood vessel, and do this every time the horse moves, for the same reason.

Pull the needle out

After all the medication has been injected, pause for a few seconds to allow the liquid to disperse into the muscle fibers, away from the needle hole. Then remove the needle with a single, smooth motion, and immediately press and massage the muscles in a circular motion to re-arrange them over the hole.

FIGURE 2.1

When giving an injection in the rump muscles, choose a site that's not horizontal, but that has a slope to aid in dispersal of the medication. Otherwise, pooling, tissue irritation, and abscess formation can result, as it did in these horses.

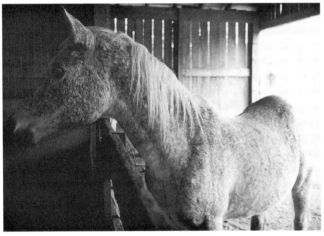

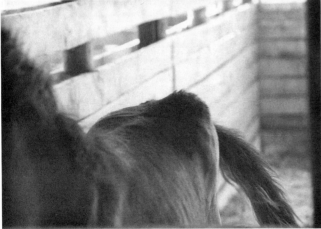

Colic

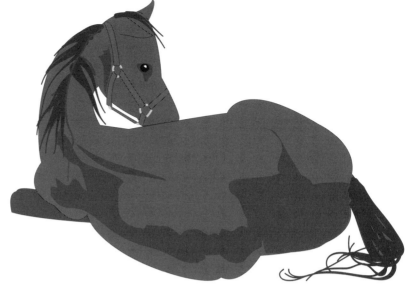

The only thing you can do if your horse colics is keep him moving and wait for the vet.

Right?

Wrong.

In the old days owners *had* to treat their own horses, because veterinary medicine, such as it was, was not available to the average horseman. But today, despite the growth of the veterinary profession, horses and horsepeople have become more mobile, and it's not uncommon for active horsepeople to find themselves, once again, in that proverbial tight spot — their horse is colicky, they're in the middle of nowhere, and there isn't an equine veterinarian for a hundred miles or more.

Many experts discourage owners from administering any treatment at all to their colicky horses, for two reasons:

1. Without proper guidance, the owner might choose the wrong treatments for his horse — the wrong drugs, the wrong dose, the wrong mode of administration — and not only fail to improve the situation but possibly make it worse.

2. A colicky horse that's been owner-treated might appear to be in less trouble than he really is, and proper veterinary treatment might therefore be delayed until it's too late to save him.

These are legitimate concerns. But what if you've been given the guidance you need, you understand that you should give only those treatments that won't mask the signs of a severe problem, your vet has entrusted you with a small, emergency cache of select medications just in case a problem arises while you're on the road, and now here you are, out in the middle of nowhere, hours away from the nearest competent equine veterinarian, and your horse is in trouble — should you *still* adhere to the unwritten rule and do nothing except find a vet? Not according to the research that's been done in the past ten years.

In colonial times, a colicky horse was "treated" by force-feeding a hornet's nest. In the late 19th century, the treatment was a drench of ammonia, raw linseed oil, turpentine, belladonna, and/or extract of cannabis (yes, marijuana) — "cures" that today would be considered poisons, or torture. In many cases, patients that survived did so in spite of, rather than because of, the treatment they received, and the only option if they didn't improve was to repeat the "cure," or shoot the horse.

In fact, thanks to that research, we've learned that early intervention in the treatment of colic is always in the best interest of the horse. That's because the key to colic survival, whether it's the kind of colic that ultimately requires surgery or not, is quick action.

So yes — if you're away from veterinary service and you're willing to accept the responsibility, you should take early interventive steps to treat your colicky horse, while simultaneously moving heaven and earth to locate a competent and willing veterinarian to take over for you as soon as possible. That way, if it turns out to be a case that will require continued and more technical care, you'll have professional help standing by, and you'll have taken steps to improve your horse's condition in the meantime to give him the best possible chance of survival.

In other words, your treatments will not substitute for veterinary care — rather, they will act as a vital prelude to it.

Why is colic painful?

Colic is painful because of pain-sensing nerves in the gut that are exquisitely sensitive to s-t-r-e-t-c-h-i-n-g of the intestinal wall due to the buildup of gas, liquid, and solids when movement through the involved loop of bowel is somehow blocked. Those same nerves are pretty blasé about other traumas, like cutting or rupturing — it's mainly the stretching of the intestinal wall that brings a horse to his knees.

Why is early intervention so important?

It isn't the colic that kills colicky horses — it's a nasty side-effect of colic called endotoxic shock. No matter what kind of colic your horse has, and no matter how it started, his body reacts to that intestinal mishap in a dangerous and predictable way:

- The flow of intestinal contents is interrupted, which causes a backup, which causes pain.
- Pain causes nearby arteries to spasm, thereby impairing blood supply to already stressed-out intestines, and continued pain eventually causes all gut motility to stop.
- This results in gas accumulating along the entire length of the intestines and even more pain.
- The troubled gut secretes inflammatory chemicals that act like fuel to a fire: they escalate the pain and speed the destruction of the troubled gut.
- The flow and absorption of liquids through the intestines is impaired, and the section of intestine at the site of the problem begins to hemorrhage. The horse becomes dehydrated, and the total volume of blood in his circulatory system

MAKE THE TOUGHEST DECISION WAY AHEAD OF TIME

Long before your horse ever colics, decide whether or not you will agree to colic surgery if it becomes necessary — in the heat of the moment, it's difficult to think clearly. Consider these points:

1. Only you know the value of your horse, and it may have nothing to do with his price tag.

2. Figure on $2500-$4000 for the surgery, depending on the specifics of your horse's case. Add pre-surgical care and aftercare, and the total bill can be more than twice the initial surgery fee, *whether or not the horse survives*.

3. Horses that have had belly surgery are statistically more likely to colic again.

4. Statistically, survival after colic surgery depends on how long the horse was colicky, the skill and experience of the surgeon, and exactly what *caused* the colic in the first place. In many cases, surgery is required to find the cause.

5. If you've got a mortality insurance policy on your horse, the decision of whether or not to give permission for surgery is not yours— the insurance company decides whether you and your horse will have to bear the expense and pain of major surgery and a precarious recovery with an uncertain future. The policy protects you against financial loss if your horse dies, but it does *not* protect you against the expense of trying to save him, even if he dies anyway, unless you get a major medical rider. If, in the heat of the moment, you decide to disobey the insurance company and have the horse euthanized, you forfeit the coverage and all those expensive premiums.

6. Whatever you decide, be sure that you tell the vet of your decision — the veterinarian you finally locate while on the road is probably a total stranger to you. It might be wrong, but it's human nature to assume that an owner with a fancy rig and nice clothes wants and can afford "the works," while a tired, raggedy-looking owner with a rusty, mismatched towing outfit is operating on a shoestring and wants a quick fix with the smallest bill possible. Talk to the vet, ask questions, get an estimate, and make your desires known.

Neither you nor any veterinarian can tell, at first, how a colic is going to turn out. To do nothing but "wait and see" if he gets better on his own is to invite him to progress to the next stage, where his condition will definitely be worse and where it will definitely be more difficult to help him.

drops (this is called *hypovolemia*).

- Meanwhile, the walls of the beleaguered intestine are beginning to deteriorate from slowed blood circulation and from pressure (gas and liquid buildup are stretching the intestine like a beach ball), and the bacteria that normally live inside the intestines begin to leak out through the damaged walls, where their endotoxins are quickly absorbed into the bloodstream.

- Now we've passed through the doorway to endotoxic shock, and with each passing moment the door is swinging closed behind us. The toxins set up a sort of massive allergic/panic reaction in the horse's circulatory system: the heart weakens, blood flow to the extremities is blocked as arteries in those areas spasm closed, and the arteries in the gut essentially go limp, allowing blood to "pool" and stagnate. The heart rate becomes rapid and weak, and the attitude changes from painful and anxious to spacy and depressed. The eyes glaze over, the gums turn a muddy, reddish-brownish color, and death is imminent.

In a recent survey, colic was the #1 concern of horse owners and the most common emergency call reported by equine veterinarians

To make matters worse, this entire sequence of events, from first sign of belly ache to irreversible, fatal shock, can take as few as four hours, depending on the specifics of the case. Whether the event that started the colic was something dramatic like a twisted gut, or something innocent like constipation, the cascade of events that follows endotoxemia is not prejudiced — the body's reaction is predictable and potentially deadly.

Now here's the good news. Even though you can't always fix the underlying problem that's plagueing your horse without a vet's help, you *can* do some things that will interrupt and slow his downslide toward endotoxic shock: you can buy him some time by protecting him from many of the circulatory consequences of endotoxemia. If it turns out that he doesn't need surgery, you'll have abbreviated his pain and cut your vet bill considerably. If he does need surgery, you'll have brought him to the surgery table in much better condition than he would have been if you hadn't intervened. Whether or not you and the vet decide that surgery is needed, your intervention means a much higher chance of survival.

Read on for a step-by-step account of how to accomplish this.

What the symptoms mean — and what they don't mean

You probably don't have any trouble recognizing the signs of colic, despite the fact that they can vary in severity from barely perceptible and subtle, to such dramatic and violent symptoms that you'd have to be blind to miss them. The trouble is, "colic" is not a diagnosis — it just means *belly pain*, and whether your horse's pain is due to a temporary backup of gas or a life-threatening twisted gut, from the outside both extremes can look the same at first. What looks like a mild colic can, in a short time, evolve into a classic thrasher — even a horse with a twisted gut can look merely "bewildered" at first. By the same token, a scary, violent looking colic can be the sort that will magically resolve with the passage of music-to-your-ears flatulence. You just can't tell, at first, how any particular colic is going to turn out, and in most cases, neither can a veterinarian — it's going to take some careful observation and a little time to make that distinction. So when your horse colics, what you see from the outside is his pain, ranging from mild to violent, but the severity of the signs does not necessarily parallel the seriousness of his problem.

The worst thing you can do is take the "wait and see" tactic when your horse's colic pain appears to be mild — mild discomfort is a gift, an opportunity to take action and reverse the problem before it snowballs, if it chooses to do so. To do nothing but "wait and see" if he gets better on his own is to invite him to progress to the next stage, where his condition will definitely be worse and where it will definitely be more difficult to help him. Furthermore, it's not at all unusual for a truly mild colic, one that fully intended to resolve on its own, to suddenly change into the kind of colic that absolutely requires surgery for any chance of survival.

There's a very logical reason for this. When a section of intestine is in distress for any reason, two things can become compromised right away: its blood supply, and its electrical system. Both must be in top working order to keep the gut functioning properly. Normal intestines move, all by themselves, like a barrel full of serpents. That movement, called intestinal motility, is how the intestinal contents get kneaded, mixed with digestive juices, and moved "downstream" toward the rectum. If there's an interruption in normal gut circulation, and/or if the electrical system begins to go haywire, the movement of the involved section of intestine can become illogical, and as a result the bowel can crawl out of position and get caught somewhere, even tie itself into a sort of knot.

So not only might your horse's colic be worse than it looks from the outside right now, it might also *become* worse than it was originally, if you don't intervene quickly enough to nip it in the bud before the gut gets itself into bigger trouble.

So should you be worried about your mildly colicky horse? Absolutely. The good news is, even though colic is alarmingly common in horses, and even though the outcome can be deadly, the vast majority of colics have happy endings — about 80% get better with just conservative treatment. But you can't afford to be complacent if your horse's case looks like "just a mild colic" — treat *all* colics as though they were dangerous and potentially life-threatening. Because they are.

What kinds of colic are there?

There are five kinds.

1. Nonstrangulating colic (bowel contents are backed up, but the blood supply to the bowel itself is still intact). This category is by far the most common, and it includes the "simple" colics, such as gut spasms, excess gas, and impactions. Definitely the kind of colic to get, if you must get any kind at all — surgery is rarely needed, and the odds of survival are the best.

2. Strangulating colic (typically a "twist," whereby both the bowel and its blood vessels have been twisted closed, not only blocking the passage of bowel contents but also pinching off the blood vessels that keep that loop of bowel alive). This is also called "accidental colic," and short of a miracle, survival is only possible (but not guaranteed) with surgery.

The entire sequence of events, from first sign of bellyache to irreversible, fatal shock, can take as few as four hours.

3. Infarction colic (bowel contents aren't physically blocked, but a blood clot has lodged in an artery supplying the involved loop of bowel, thereby "suffocating" it — the bowel stops moving because its blood supply has been cut off). Surgery is only needed when the blocked blood vessel is a big one, resulting in a piece of intestine actually dying (instead of just getting "sick" temporarily until neighboring blood vessels manage to pick up the circulatory slack).

4. Enteritis (the intestine has become "sick" from an inflammatory process, such as an infection). Surgery is definitely not needed in this kind of colic, although exploratory surgery is sometimes done just to figure out what's causing the horse's problem — and the stress of the anesthesia and surgery can hasten his demise.

5. Overeating colic (the horse gets into the grain supply and stuffs himself with grain). This is no joke. The sudden glut of grain causes a population explosion in gut bacteria, and those bacteria release an overwhelming dose of toxins that cause a *rapidly fatal* endotoxic shock.

What causes colic?

Because of the way a horse is designed — a digestive tract that's nearly 100 feet long, all crammed into a relatively small space — the odds are stacked against him as far as colic is concerned. But recent studies have shown that certain external factors can affect your horse's chances of falling victim to this uniquely equine disease. For example:

- Parasites (worms) and the damage they do to the intestines and their blood supply are a major cause of colic.
- The more time a horse spends in a trailer, the greater is the risk of colic.
- Horses used in competitions and in race training have significantly more colic than horses in other activities.
- Horses with access to pasture have less colic than horses kept in stalls or drylots.
- Horses on a daily deworming program have a much lower colic risk than horses given purge-dewormers every six to eight weeks.
- Horses cared for by a trainer or a manager are three or two times, respectively, more likely to colic than horses cared for by their owners.
- Colic is most common in Arabians, followed by Warmbloods, then Thoroughbreds, then Quarter Horses, then Standardbreds, and mixed-breed horses have the lowest incidence.

- Horses between the ages of two to ten years have the highest incidence of colic.
- A very serious type of surgical colic known as torsion of the colon is much more common in broodmares within two months after foaling than in any other horses.
- Contrary to popular belief, colic is not linked to abrupt changes in the weather.

No doubt about it, worms cause a lot of colics. Stongyle-type worms can damage and plug the blood vessels that feed the intestines, pinching off the blood supply just a little bit — enough to affect the gut's electrical system — or cutting it off entirely, causing a section of intestine to die from lack of blood. Tapeworms can cause cauliflower-like growths in the gut, jutting belligerently into the flow of traffic and causing all kinds of trouble. Other worms simply dam the intestines like a tangle of spaghetti.

The severity of the pain does not necessarily indicate the seriousness of the colic.

Performance horses are especially prone to impactions and twists. Perhaps that's because their diet when on the road lacks sufficient fiber to keep the guts working properly (because they're less bulky and easier to carry, low-fiber pelleted feeds are often brought along instead of the usual hay and grain). Or perhaps it's because they don't like to drink the "foreign" water away from home. And even if your horse is meticulously dewormed, parasites can be a problem when on the road if he's turned out in a public paddock that's loaded with worm eggs from hundreds of wormy horses that have spent an hour or two in that same paddock over the years. If your horse spends just an hour or two in that paddock, he can pick up *millions* of larvae, and seven days later, when those larvae molt and release an irritating chemical, your horse's gut lining can become inflamed and raw, and *voila!*— he's got colic. Another hazard in borrowed paddocks is toxic weeds — exhausted and very hungry after spending the day in a trailer, your horse might eat things he wouldn't ordinarily consider.

Performance horses are especially prone to colic.

The most pervasive colic factor in performance horses is stress — the stress of separation from herd buddies, fatigue, performance anxiety, diet and watering changes, mixing with strange horses, and whiffing their potpourri of germs.

Why is colic so dangerous?

It's hard for people to understand that colic, an intestinal condition, kills by affecting the heart and lungs, but that's exactly what happens.

It can begin innocently enough, with a backup of liquid and/or gas from some sort of internal traffic jam. As the liquids and gases accumulate, the bowel becomes distended, which is excruciatingly painful, and the pressure can build to the point that it rivals a fully inflated basketball. It pushes against the diaphragm, compressing the chest and making it difficult to breathe. The rest of the intestines react to the pain and pressure by at first speeding up (thereby trying to "blast" the obstruction away), then slowing, and eventually stopping all motility. Now, since *nothing* is moving, gas accumulates along the *entire* length of the intestinal tract.

The troubled intestines release chemicals called arachidonic acid metabolites (from now on, I'll call them "caustic chemicals"). These chemicals cause important blood vessels in the body to constrict, depriving the heart, lungs, and extremities of blood, while at the same time escalating the pain and intestinal damage. This process is aided and abetted by endotoxins released by the bacteria in the intestines, further damaging the heart and lungs. As the intestinal walls deteriorate, the endotoxins and caustic chemicals leak through the damaged areas and are absorbed into the bloodstream, pulling the horse toward the point of no return: endotoxic shock.

If your horse's colic involves a **"twist,"** the involved intestine deteriorates even faster than in the nonstrangulating types of colic because the twist cuts off its blood supply. The gut begins to hemorrhage and swell, causing massive blood loss, the release of the caustic chemicals, severe pain, and the absorption of endotoxins. In this kind of colic, endotoxic shock can develop so quickly that the horse can sink past the point of no return within four to six hours.

In **infarction colic**, which starts with a blood clot from migrating strongyle larvae, the involved artery does exactly the wrong thing: it spasms, essentially finishing the job started by the clot, making sure that no blood can get past the blockage. There won't exactly be a physical obstruction inside the intestine at that point, *but the intestine will stop moving*, thanks to its blood supply being cut off. The result is a functional blockage: nothing will be able to move through the involved loop, because it's "unconscious." Gas builds up, stretching the walls of the intestine, and pain sets the now familiar, deadly cascade of events into motion: the bowel wall starts to degenerate, bacteria and their toxins are absorbed, and the horse heads down the lane toward endotoxic shock.

Ironically, some of the milder cases of infarction colic aren't "colics" at all — if it's a very small artery that's been blocked, there may initially be *no pain*. But because of the glitch in the circulation caused by the blood clot, the involved intestine's electrical system starts going haywire, and the intestine gets "confused," moving illogically out of place and getting itself into trouble. *Now* you've got classic colic pain. This horse might make it to the surgeon's table in time, and the surgeon might skillfully put the errant loop of bowel back into its rightful place — but of course this didn't really address the original problem, which was an alteration in blood flow. You guessed it, this horse is likely to colic again, and very soon, unless somebody recognizes and corrects his worm problem.

In **enteritis**, instead of being blocked or twisted, the intestines are severely inflamed, usually because of an infection such as Salmonellosis. The infection shuts down the gut motility, gas accumulates and there may be no manure passed at all while the intestinal lining slowly "catches fire" and erodes. This erosion allows bacteria and their endotoxins to leak through the raw, irritated tissues and enter the bloodstream. The pain, which looks just like any other kind of colic, changes to a

Surgery might "cure" the immediate colic without addressing what caused it to happen in the first place, such as worm damage. Colic is likely to recur in such cases unless the underlying problem is found and corrected.

stuporous depression, and *then* you get your first obvious sign of what's going on: the horse develops *diarrhea*. By this time, endotoxic shock is well under way. Hospitalization and intensive care are required for any chance of survival, and survivors are prime candidates for founder.

In **overeating colic**, high doses of endotoxin are absorbed into the bloodstream from bacteria feasting on the gluttonous meal, and the result is endotoxic shock. From the outside it looks like this: abdominal pain, no gut sounds, rapid heart rate, rapid shallow breathing, pale gums, prolonged capillary refill time, and finally diarrhea and death. Fast treatment (given when you suspect that the horse has overeaten but he doesn't look "sick" yet) can prevent the endotoxemia, but horses that are treated after they become endotoxemic are practically guaranteed to founder (see *Chapter 5*).

What Would the Vet Do?

A sharp equine veterinarian would simultaneously

1. gather all the data available to help narrow down the cause of the colic,

2. administer treatments to make the horse more comfortable,

3. prevent, block, and/or reverse the destructive cascade of events leading to inflammation and endotoxic shock, and

4. resolve the underlying problem — or — make the decision to ship the horse to a surgeon as early in the course of the colic as possible.

Ideally, the horse would be re-assessed frequently (i.e., every ten to fifteen minutes) during the course of treatment to see how he's responding, to decide whether different and/or additional treatment is needed, and to see if the initial diagnostic impressions should be adjusted. Any treatments that might change the horse's symptoms and mislead diagnostic efforts would be given only *after* the appropriate observations had been made. Furthermore, no treatment that might be good for one type of colic but bad for another type would be given until the vet is relatively certain that the treatment will do no harm.

This is the ideal, and in this ideal, the vet would stay with the horse for at least an hour, often longer — checking, administering, re-checking, administering some more, re-checking — gradually refining his/her diagnosis, meeting all of the horse's needs to maintain optimal overall condition during treatment, while approaching a meaningful prediction about whether or not surgery will be needed.

The veterinarian has many tools and skills at his/her disposal that you don't have, including rectal palpation, the passage of a stomach tube, ultrasound technology, laboratory tests, the "belly tap," and, perhaps most important of all in a crisis where time is of the essence, *experience*.

SPECIAL NOTE 3.1

DSS (dioctyl sodium sulfosuccinate), sold in various over-the-counter products as a "stool softener," is touted by some as a layperson's alternative to having a horse "tubed" with mineral oil because of its smaller volume and the fact that some commercial preparations are available in handy paste-syringes. However, there are numerous reports of DSS causing colic and diarrhea in horses. Don't use it in your horse unless your vet approves.

POST-COLIC FOUNDER

Early signs of founder (also known as laminitis) include heat in one or more feet (usually, but not always, the front feet), with an obvious digital pulse in the involved feet. Stiffness, lameness, and/or the classic "sawhorse stance" appear soon afterward. For more on founder, including how to check the feet for excess heat and a digital pulse, as well as what to do about it if you suspect your horse is foundering, see *Chapter 5 (Founder)* and *Chapter 19 (Vital Signs)*.

WHEN IS A MOLEHILL REALLY A MOUNTAIN?

Let's say your horse's colic is a truly mild one, a temporary buildup of gas. The gas is doing its best to navigate around a tight bend, but it's accumulating faster than it can pass. Once it passes, which it should eventually be able to do, everything will be fine. But the pain is causing spasms in nearby blood vessels, which is impairing the circulation to the gut, and it's also causing some caustic chemicals to ooze from the walls of the intestine, further irritating the already troubled tissues. As a result, an electrical problem — a "short," if you will, begins to develop.

As is often the case when gas first starts to build, the motility of the gut increases in an attempt to "blast through" the problem — this period of increased motility can last as long as two hours. Meanwhile the electrical "short" is spreading and beginning to affect the guts' movements. So now the guts, which were moving in a frantic but *logical* manner, begin to move *illogically*.

To make matters worse, equine intestines are not firmly anchored into their proper place, and the streamlined, built-for-speed equine chassis has very little room for error inside the abdomen. Therefore, if a loop of bowel wanders out of position, which it might do if its electrical system has gone haywire, chances are very good that it will soon be pinned down by adjacent organs. It might even twist over itself, or tie itself into a sort of knot. It's a classsic case of the body responding to a problem in a self-defeating way. In this situation, if left to her own devices, Mother Nature will kill your horse. Your intervention can make all the difference.

If it's the sort of colic that requires surgery from the git-go, your efforts can, at the very least, stabilize his general condition by controlling the pain and all the self-destructive ways in which the body responds to it, by blocking the action of the inflammatory chemicals produced by the troubled intestine, and by blocking and actually reversing some of the effects of endotoxins being absorbed through the damaged intestinal wall. At the very least, you'll improve the odds that your horse will survive the general anesthesia and the significant stress of surgery.

There's No Vet — What Should You Do?

There are two ground rules you must follow in treating your horse for colic. The number one ground rule also applies to veterinarians: DO NO HARM. The specific treatment for your horse's colic will depend on which of the five kinds of colic he has: strangulating, nonstrangulating, infarction, enteritis, or overeating. By following the step-by-step formula in the Colic Procedure Checklist below, you'll start the narrowing-down process and maybe even figure out which kind of colic your horse has. If so, great — you will have come that much closer to knowing exactly what your horse needs in order to resolve this colic, you'll have a lot more treatment options than if you don't have any idea what's causing his problem, and by passing your observations on to the referral vet, you will help to shortcut the diagnostic process. But if you can't make any progress in figuring it out, that's okay too — you'll simply have to limit your treatment approach so that you can do some good without the risk of making the situation worse.

The other ground rule applies only to you: while tending to your horse's immediate needs, you must simultaneously be working on getting your horse within reach of a competent equine veterinarian who can take over for you — even if you just park in the clinic's parking lot with your cellular phone warmed up and ready to call. You can do a great deal to help your horse by yourself, but there are many things, both diagnostically and therapeutically, that only a vet can do. Don't make your horse wait any longer for professional help than is absolutely necessary.

Are you ready to get started? Here we go, one step at a time....

THE COLIC PROCEDURE CHECKLIST

The following checklist can guide you through the first two hours of a colic. While following these steps, you should also be in the process of securing veterinary backup to confirm your horse's full recovery and check for an underlying cause, or to resume treatment in case he does not respond completely within the time period outlined in this checklist. Accordingly, just in case a blockage persists even though the horse appears improved, it is not recommended to resume full feed until the horse has passed at least five normal manure piles (about three gallons of manure).

If, during the course of this checklist, any of the following signs appears, consider the need for veterinary assistance to be urgent and mandatory:

- green froth coming from the nostrils
- worsening vital signs
- persistent or escalating pain despite treatment with Banamine™
- rectal temperature dropping below 99ºF
- diarrhea
- laminitis
- any clues suggesting that the colic started with a grain overload

time	√	procedure
00:00	√	Grade the pain (see *The Pain Gauge*, page 31)
	√	Check vital signs (see *Special Note 3.2*)
	√	Write it down (keep a detailed diary of findings and procedures — the referral vet will find the information helpful).

time	√	procedure

00:15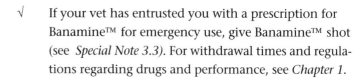

√ If your vet has entrusted you with a prescription for Banamine™ for emergency use, give Banamine™ shot (see *Special Note 3.3*). For withdrawal times and regulations regarding drugs and performance, see *Chapter 1.*

√ If pain ≥ level 4, also provide protective head gear (see *Chapter 18*).

√ If signs of laminitis/founder are present (hot feet, digital pulse, lameness), or if horse has fever ≥ 101.5ºF or diarrhea, or if anything about this case suggests enteritis or overeating colic, AND if there is no green froth at nostrils, and you have a presciption for it, also give phenylbutazone ("bute") paste or gel orally (see *Special Note 3.5)*, affix wedges to heels (see *Chapter 5, Founder)*, and do not move the horse any more than is absolutely necessary. DO NOT ATTEMPT TO GIVE INJECTABLE BUTE. Refer to *Chapter 5* for more on care of the foundering horse. For withdrawal times and regulations regarding drugs and performance, see *Chapter 1.*

√ Write it all down.

00:20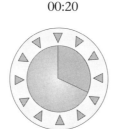

√ Confine horse to clean area where manure output can be monitored and feed intake restricted. From now until the case is either referred or resolved, collect all manure the horse passes and examine it as described (see *Special Note 3.4).*

√ Remove all edible bedding if the horse seems intent on nibbling, and remove all feed except as instructed later in this checklist.

√ Give colic enema (see *Special Note 3.10).*

√ Write down time, amount, and results of exam on all manure passed.

SPECIAL NOTE 3.3

BANAMINE™ DOSE FOR COLIC

800 lb horse:	3 cc
900 lb horse:	3 cc
1,000 lb horse:	3-1/2 cc
1,100 lb horse:	4 cc
1,200 lb horse:	4 cc
1,300 lb horse:	4-1/2 cc
1,400 lb horse:	5 cc

To be given intramuscularly, once only.

SPECIAL NOTE 3.4

MANURE CHECK:

Examine all manure passed for volume, color, consistency, abnormal odor (some manure smells extra "foul" or sour), and for foreign bodies such as twine, hardware, wood, etc. Also check for sand: Thoroughly mix one or two manure balls in a clear glass jar full of warm water, then set aside and let stand for 30 min. Lift jar and look through the bottom: any sand will have settled there. Be sure to report the results of this test to any referral veterinarian you see for this colic.

THE PAIN GAUGE

PAIN	level 1	level 2	level 3	level 4	level 5
QUALITY	Subtle.	Mild.	Moderate.	Violent.	Shock.
ATTITUDE	Quiet.	Confused, preoccupied, but will pay attention if interrupted.	Fixated on pain, distraught, can be interrupted but has very short attention span.	Possessed, rabid with pain, aware of nothing else but the pain.	"Out of it," oblivious, in a stupor, difficult or impossible to distract.
EXPRESSION	Sleepy.	Restless.	Anxious.	Panicked.	Dazed.
DIRECT SYMPTOMS	Yawning.	Pawing the ground, wringing the tail, looking at sides, stretching neck, curling lip.	Sweating, crouching as if preparing to lie down, stretching, kicking at belly, biting at flanks.	Crashing to the ground.	An eerie sort of surrender.
POSITION	Standing or lying quietly.	Up and down.	Occasionally rolling.	Thrashing.	Usually down, very difficult to arouse.

time	√	procedure

00:30   √   Grade the pain

√   Check vital signs (see *Special Note 3.2*)

√   If pain &/or vital signs have shown no improvement by now, or have worsened in spite of treatment, give second dose of Banamine™. Note that this second dose might mask signs of endotoxemia. The referral veterinarian *must* be made aware that you have given this.

√   Write it down

SPECIAL NOTE 3.5

BUTE DOSE FOR COLIC

800 lb horse:	1 gram
900 lb horse:	1 gram
1,000 lb horse:	1 gram
1,100 lb horse:	1-1/2 grams
1,200 lb horse:	1-1/2 grams
1,300 lb horse:	1-1/2 grams
1,400 lb horse:	2 grams

To be given orally, once only, if founder is suspected.

time	√	procedure

00:35   √   From now until the case is either referred or resolved, if pain ≤ level 3 and there are/were no signs of founder, walk the horse 5 min every hour, leading up and down gentle slopes if possible. Do not force horses with pain levels of 4 or 5 to walk.

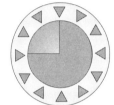

SPECIAL NOTE 3.6

A horse with severe colic pain can be violent and self destructive, crashing to the ground and risking concussion, eye injury, fractures, abrasions and lacerations. For his and your safety, put him where there are no obstacles or protrusions. Also, if you can do so safely, pad his head with a "crash helmet" (see *Chapter 18*) to protect his eyes and absorb concussion. Remove all buckets, hooks, and other potential hazards, cushion the floor with heavy bedding, and line the walls with bales of straw (a horse this painful is not likely to eat the bedding).

00:45   √   Grade the pain

  √   Check vital signs

  √   Write it down

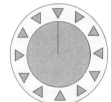

00:60   √   Grade the pain

  √   Check vital signs

  √   Write it down

01:05   √   If pain ≤ level 3 and has not escalated over the past hour, and if there is no green froth at nostrils, offer two 1-gallon buckets of water side-by-side: one with added electrolyte powder, one plain. Water should be cool — not cold or warm. Record what and how much he drinks and replenish and/or refresh often.

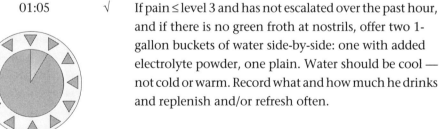

SPECIAL NOTE 3.7

THE PSYLLIUM MASH

Psyllium is a laxative that draws water into the gut and stimulates gut motility. Obviously a laxative would be the wrong thing to give if it has no chance of pushing through; therefore, the psyllium mash is to be given only when the pain has been ≤ level 1 for at least 2 hours and at least 2 gallons of manure have passed within the past hour *after* the rectum was cleaned out with an enema — with few exceptions, a horse with an intestinal impasse would be unlikely to meet these criteria (see *Special Note 3.9*).

THE RECIPE:

1 cup whole or crimped oats
2 teaspoons loose salt
4 Tablespoons equine psyllium product
1/4 cup liquid molasses
1 chopped apple (optional)
1 cup wheat bran (optional)
1/2 cup hot water (less or more as needed to make pleasant consistency)

Mix ingredients well; add small amounts water or bran as needed to make a pleasant consistency.

time	√	procedure

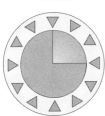

01:15   √   If pain ≤ level 1 and has not escalated over the past hour, at least 2 gallons of manure have passed since you cleaned him out with the enema, and if there is no green froth at nostrils, offer one dose PSYLLIUM MASH (see *Special Note 3.7*). Record the time and his response.

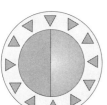

01:30   √   Grade the pain

        √   Check vital signs

        √   Write it down

SPECIAL NOTE 3.8

There are many good equine electrolyte products for use in drinking water. Choose one that is meant for adult horses (not for calves with diarrhea), and mix it according to the instructions on the label. Always offer a bucket of untreated (plain) water at the same time.

time	√	procedure

01:45 √ Grade the pain

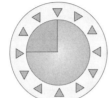 √ Check vital signs

√ Write it down

SPECIAL NOTE 3.9

What does it mean if the colicky horse passes manure? Maybe nothing — he can "hoard" up to two gallons in his rectum, so what he passes might only be a "stash" from earlier in the day. Anything over two gallons, though, is probably significant. The biggest danger in a horse with dull, mild, but persistent colic pain is cecal impaction — he might continue to eat, which will just add to the impaction. That's why it's important to give an enema early in the course of the colic — to empty out his rectum so you can interpret any voluntary bowel movements that occur after the enema has cleaned him out.

Decision time

02:00 √ If you aren't absolutely sure that he's absolutely normal by now, you're in over your head. If you haven't already arranged for a veterinarian to meet you and aren't already on the road to his/her equine veterinary facility, get going.

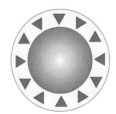

√ If he seems fine now and you've gotten at least 2 gallons of manure out *after* he finished defecating from the enema, feed the following restricted diet until 3 more gallons have passed: 1 shoebox hay every hour, 1 oil mash every 3 hours (See recipe at left). Continue checking pain and vital signs regularly. Any resurgence of pain is *bad news.* Be well positioned to get to your referral vet fast. (No more pain killers are warranted.)

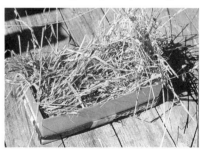

THE OIL MASH

1 cup whole or crimped oats
1 cup wheat bran
1/4 cup liquid molasses
1 cup mineral oil
1 sliced apple

THE SHOEBOX OF HAY
It's as simple as it sounds: it's enough grass hay to loosely fill a standard shoebox.

SPECIAL NOTE 3.10

THE COLIC ENEMA

Materials:

Reusable 2-quart capacity, balloon-type feminine douche bag
2 cups mineral oil
warm tap water
lubricating jelly

Pour mineral oil into the bag, pinching the neck as needed to open the one-way valve so the oil will enter. Press the bag against the faucet and fill, under pressure, so it "balloons," to approximately 1 quart of total contents.

Liberally lubricate the end of the catheter portion and insert into the horse's rectum. Attach the bag and hold the apparatus in place while the liquid flows into the rectum. If possible, do not hold the horse's tail, as this will only draw attention to what you're doing and encourage him to start pushing sooner. As the bag empties, the liquid might flow more slowly — it's okay to squeeze the bag a little to speed things up a bit. Remove the apparatus when all the liquid has been delivered.

Collect all solids and add to manure bucket.

If your horse's condition improves with your treatment and you decide not to seek veterinary backup, make this judgment at your own risk — he's not necessarily out of the woods yet, because you don't know what caused him to colic in the first place.

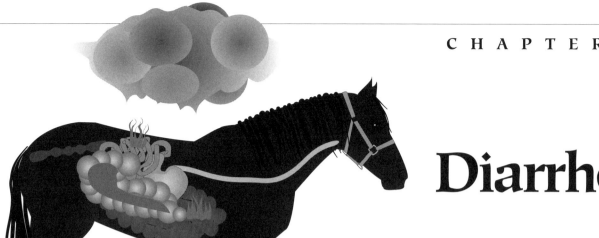

Diarrhea

The sudden onset of diarrhea — true diarrhea — in an adult horse is never anything less than an emergency. It might be cause for only moderate alarm in a youngster, in which the physiologic events that cause it are more common. But when a foal matures into a full-grown adult, he leaves behind the tendency for such intestinal shenanigans. If diarrhea strikes your adult horse, you should become immediately alarmed.

What you see

There's a big difference between diarrhea and loose stool. Loose stool, which can result from such benign influences as temporary nervousness, is an excessively watery bowel movement that occurs at the same or slightly higher frequency than normal bowel movements. In other words, he isn't "going" significantly more often than usual, it's just coming out wetter.

Diarrhea, however, is characterized not only by excessive water in the stool, but also by a significant increase in the frequency of bowel movements. This should be evident in the environment —there are splashes of soupy manure everywhere. Instead of his usual 4 or 5 pile-output for a night's "work," for example, there's evidence of 12 or more movements. You might also notice that the manure doesn't have its usual pleasant, earthy aroma but smells soured and fermented, or more like dog feces.

In most cases, along with diarrhea, the horse might also show signs of general malaise: a droopy, depressed demeanor, lack of appetite, and fever (although fever is often missing if the diarrhea is the result of poisoning instead of an infection). Colic (nonspecific belly pain) is another common finding regardless of the diarrhea's underlying cause.

Why is this dangerous?

With all due respect to the equine species, *hayburner* is an apt nickname — horses are mostly digestive tracts, and the rest of their bodily functions (lungs, legs, brains, reproductive tracts) are secondary. The digestive tract in the horse is over 100 feet long, with its surface area being an impressive multiple of that length. When this mass of tissue becomes inflamed, the majority of the horse is inflamed. It's major, serious stuff.

The inflammatory process in the horse is prone to excess, and this is particularly true when that inflammation is occurring in the digestive tract. Caustic chemicals are secreted in response to the initial phases of inflammation, their role being to perpetuate the inflammation — to add fuel to the fire, so to speak. The result is a virtual erosion of delicate tissues whose job it is to re-absorb the 35 gallons of water moving past them within the large intestines. Those 35 gallons were "borrowed" from the bloodstream in the small intestine as a normal part of the digestive process, with the promise that as soon as the slurry of digesta reaches the large intestine, the water will be reabsorbed and the debt will be repaid.

In the old days, diarrhea was treated with drugs to stop the flow of manure. Today we recognize that the diarrhea is occurring for a reason, and the focus is on supporting the bodily functions while the diarrhea runs its course.

But in diarrhea, two things can go wrong. First of all, the amount of water borrowed in the small intestine can escalate way beyond the usual 35 gallons, because when the small intestines are irritated they ooze. This is called *secretory diarrhea* because a major portion of the too-juicy manure comes from the liquids secreted in the small intestine.

To make matters worse, when the digesta reach the large intestine, suddenly the large intestine's ability to re-absorb that water so it can be returned to the circulatory system is impaired, either because the lining of the large intestine is irritated and swollen (*colitis*) or because the digesta are screaming through there so fast that the absorption simply can't take place quickly enough (*hypermotility*).

The result is a rapid and profound upset of the horse's water and electrolyte balance, and, depending on how rapidly it takes place, it can be life threatening before the day is over.

What would the vet do?

The sharp veterinarian would refrain from reflexly administering "diarrhea medications" until he/she had narrowed down the cause of your horse's problem. The treatment for *inflammatory* diarrhea (enteritis, colitis) is different than the treatment for *secretory* or *hypermotile* or *malabsorptive* diarrhea, and if the diarrhea is due to a derangement in the gut's circulation, the treatment might focus entirely on the cause

of *that* derangement and virtually ignore what's coming out under the tail. Furthermore, the vet's actions should also hinge on whether it appears that your horse's case
is the result of a "bug" that might threaten neighboring horses (such as *Salmonella*,
E. coli, or Potomac Horse Fever), a poisonous substance (such as blister beetles,
buttercups, fly spray, or moldy feed), or the "mystery disease" *Colitis-X*.

In the old days, treatment was aimed at stopping the flow of manure:
medications were given that would practically paralyze the gut's motility so that the
flow of digesta would stop or at least significantly slow down. Today the focus is on
supporting the body in the hope that the diarrhea will stop itself — rather than stop
the flow of digesta and essentially trap infectious organisms, endotoxins, inflammatory chemicals, and poisons inside the horse where they can do more damage, let
them come out, but help the horse by keeping him hydrated, keeping his electrolytes
from being depleted, and trying to moderate the inflammation that's burning out of
control. And, of course, if the underlying cause has been determined, it is also
addressed.

So the sharp veterinarian would

- run laboratory tests to identify any infectious organisms causing the illness,
- correct and maintain the horse's hydration and electrolyte balance,
- administer an antiinflammatory/antiprostaglandin/antiendotoxin/anti-fe
  ver medication such as Banamine™ if indicated,
- administer upper gi soothants/protectants (such as Kaopectate™ or mineral oil or
  Pepto-Bismol™) to slow down its excessive secretion,
- administer an antidote if the horse was poisoned and an antidote is available,
- administer antibiotics and probiotics if a bacterial cause is suspected,
- institute a quarantine if appropriate (and, if required, report his/her suspicions of
  Salmonellosis or Potomac Horse Fever to authorities), and
- take steps to prevent founder, a common sequel to diarrhea.

There's no vet. What should you do?

The following steps apply only if your horse has true diarrhea, not just temporary
loose stool.

STEP 1.
Get help

No matter how long it will take, send someone to find a good equine vet who can
come to your horse's aid — at the very least, he's likely to need IV fluids. Meanwhile,
isolate him until the cause of his diarrhea is determined to be non-contagious.

STEP 2.
Check T-P-R

While you're waiting, check his rectal temperature, pulse, and respiratory rate (see
Chapter 19: Vital Signs) and write them down. Elevated vital signs can indicate
inflammation, infection, and endotoxemia. The veterinarian who accepts your case

will want to know what the initial vitals were, since they'll be affected by treatment and might, therefore, be misleading.

Listen to his gut sounds (see *Chapter 19: Vital Signs*) and write down whether your impression is that the gut is unusually quiet, normal, or excessively noisy. If it's excessively noisy, try to characterize the sounds: do you hear a lot of long growling, or does it sound juicy and gurgly, or is there a lot of gassy pinging? The vet will want this information to evaluate the horse's progress.

STEP 3.
Listen to the gut

Find out whether any other horses in your fellow's associates have recently had a similar problem, which could indicate that this is a contagious disease. Check your horse's vaccination history: has he been vaccinated against Potomac Horse Fever? If so, when? Have you recently treated chewed fenceboards with any chemicals? Used a new fly repellant on your horse? Gotten new feed? When was the last time he was dewormed? With what? Is he currently taking any antibiotics? If so, write down what he's taking, how much, and for what purpose — some antibiotics can leave a horse susceptible to infection with Salmonellosis, and others can cause Colitis X, a rapidly fatal condition. Unless directed otherwise by the referral veterinarian, stop the antibiotics — they could be killing your horse.

STEP 4.
Start the detective work

"Ask" your horse how he feels. Is he interested in his usual feeds? (If he is, don't let him have much — just a handful. You're not feeding him, you're just finding out if he's got a normal appetite). Is he showing the usual brightness, alertness, and level of interest in his surroundings, or does he seem detached and maybe even depressed? Write this down.

STEP 5.
Check for malaise

Offer three 5-gallon buckets of fresh, room-temperature water:

- one plain,
- one treated with your powdered electrolyte product according to the directions on the label (make sure it contains potassium), and
- one containing 1/3 lb (1/3 of a one pound box) of baking soda.

STEP 6.
Offer water and electrolytes

This will provide him with ready sources of all the electrolytes he might be lacking, and if he feels well enough to drink on his own, he's likely to choose the solutions that best suit his needs.
If your commercial electrolyte doesn't contain any potassium or potassium chloride, add a fourth bucket containing

- one gallon of water and five of the 3-1/8 oz canisters of Morton's Salt Substitute (it's potassium chloride).

If he's so sick that he's refusing to drink or eat, he needs intravenous fluids and electrolytes. The combination of diarrhea (massive losses) with refusal to replace those losses is a deadly one.

STEP 7.
If you're not able to get the help you need...

If no vet can be found, you'll have to make some difficult decisions on your own.

7a.
Consider giving Banamine™

- Treatment with the antiinflammatory Banamine™, for example, might help the horse a great deal by relieving his colic pain, dampening his internal inflammatory fire, and making him feel sufficiently better that he'll drink on his own. However, if your horse has been "on" Bute or Banamine for some other problem, such as a chronic lameness, for more than just a few days and still has it in his system, the last thing he needs is another dose — the drug might actually be part of his problem. Otherwise, it's a logical choice, and if your vet has entrusted you with a prescription, you should follow the dosage regimen outlined in *Chapter 3: Colic*.

7b.
Give a probiotic

- There's no safe way to recommend any antibiotic in a case of diarrhea that hasn't had its underlying cause diagnosed: the best antibiotic for Potomac Horse Fever, for example, is the worst one for Salmonellosis. What you can do, however, is try to give the "good" bacteria a boost by giving the horse a dose of an equine probiotic product. There are several commercial probiotic products available for equine use. Follow the dosage recommendations on the label.

7c.
If he has a fever, reduce it

Meanwhile, be working on trying to get his fever down (if applicable) low enough so he'll feel better and be more inclined to drink voluntarily. See page 153.

7d.
Attend to any factors interfering with your efforts at rehydrating him

Similarly, if he has serious colic pain, this will have to be alleviated before he'll take anything orally (see *Chapter 3: Colic*). Replenish and/or refresh his water buckets often so he'll be more inclined to partake. Give him no grain, but offer ten-minute sessions of grass grazing if available, or just enough grass hay to fill a standard shoebox, separating each tiny meal by half an hour.

7e.
Keep nagging him about fluids

If your horse is not drinking very well, try offering some loose salt to lick from your hand or his feed tray, or gently poke some salt directly onto the inside of his lower lip. The saltiness might stimulate his thirst.

7f.
Consider founder

Since founder is a common sequel to diarrhea, keep a close watch on your horse's feet for signs of trouble and take preventive steps if you have reason to believe it's necessary (see *Chapter 5: Founder*).

20 to 30% of all Potomac Horse Fever sufferers end up with founder.

Founder

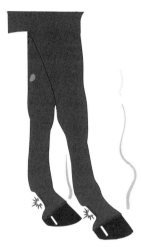

Oh no... not the "F" word. Even if you've never seen it before, you recognize it on sight: The stiff, painful forehand gait. The sawhorse stance. The hot hooves, the bounding digital pulse. It's a nightmare...this can't be happening...my beautiful horse is *ruined*..

Not necessarily. Act fast, act appropriately, ignore the well-meaning but misguided advice of "horsey" friends who tell you to "walk him out of it," and the odds are good that your beautiful horse will recover completely, or very near to it. That's what this chapter is for: to get you safely through the crisis, to help you avoid the pitfalls, and to help you do everything you can to halt the breakdown process in its tracks, so that when you finally locate a veterinarian to take over, the fire in your horse's feet will already have been contained.

Founder, also known as laminitis, is a serious, potentially life-threatening breakdown of the supporting structures inside a horse's feet. It is most often seen in the front feet but all four feet may be involved, or it might attack one foot when it's bearing excess weight to compensate for lameness in another foot.

What confuses a lot of people, and what causes dangerous delays in diagnosis and treatment, is the fact that the real problem is likely to have nothing at all to do with feet — founder is a symptom, not a disease. And as you can see in *Special Note 5.1*, some of the most common triggers of founder are occupational hazards in the performance horse.

What makes founder so potentially devastating is that it's not dependent on that underlying problem to keep it going — once it's gotten started, founder takes on a life of its own, and the cascade of destructive events inside the stricken horse's feet can become like a speeding train. It's much easier, and much more likely to be successful, to stop the thing before it really gets rolling.

What makes founder so potentially devastating is that it's not dependent on its underlying cause to keep it going — once it's gotten started, founder takes on a life of its own, and the cascade of destructive events inside the stricken horse's feet can become like a speeding train.

Confusion: founder's biggest ace in the hole

How can my horse be foundered? He doesn't fit the stereotype — he's not fat, and he doesn't get any grain at all!

Well, it's true that obesity is one of the most common causes of founder, and a diet that's heavy on grain (or a late-night raid of the grain room) is another familiar prelude to founder. But the scary truth is, because of the way the horse is put together, founder can be the result of just about any form of major stress, whether that stress be diet, illness, fever, injury, mismanagement, overwork, or something going on inside the horse that you never identify. Regardless of the underlying cause, the signs of founder are pretty much unmistakable — they vary only in severity — so don't let your confusion stand in the way of helping your horse. Stop that train now, while you still can.

Should I just have him put down?

The odds of a complete recovery depend on several things: how long the symptoms were present before treatment was started, how severe the pain is, how many feet are affected, whether or not you're able to identify (and eliminate) an underlying cause, whether or not the supportive internal structures of the foot have already begun to break down, the body weight of the horse (see *Special Note 5.2*), whether or not the coffin bone (the wedge-shaped bone inside the foot) becomes infected, and whether you're able to separate what you really should do from what well-meaning but misinformed horse buddies will tell you — like any complicated, devastating disease, founder is deeply marinated in myth, and there's a lot of advice floating around out there that can make things much, much worse.

What you see

The most reliable sign is the presence of a digital pulse, which is normally very faint and difficult to feel — about the same intensity as your own pulse at your wrist, which, as you can imagine, would be tough to find consistently on a hairy, impatient equine leg.

Place your index and middle fingers gently against the skin at the pulse points: they're at the back and slightly to the outside below each fetlock joint (see *Figure 5.4*). To get your fingers situated close to the skin, you may need to work them back and forth a bit so they can get underneath the hair. Now hold your breath and just let your fingertips *feel*.

In the normal horse, the pulse should be very faint and hard to appreciate. In the foundered horse, the pulse is stronger (but not necessarily faster) — it "bumps" your fingers a little harder and is therefore easier to feel. If you're able to feel a strong digital pulse in your horse's feet, and the hooves feel warm or hot to the touch, and he's showing signs of being tenderfooted in the forefeet, he's foundered.

How bad is it?

In the early stages it can be very subtle, but it tends to progress rather rapidly. The easiest way to assess the severity of your horse's founder is to grade his symptoms on a scale of I (mild) to III (severe):

Mild founder
GRADE I

He walks readily, and at first he might show lameness only when walked on a hard surface and/or when turned in a circle: his gait will be a little stiff and stilted, a little hesitant. When standing at rest he may act a bit restless, as though the floor is hot, frequently shifting his weight from foot to foot every few seconds. His attitude might be a bit lethargic, his appetite picky, and he might appear preoccupied. If you try to lift one foot, he gives it to you readily, with no hesitation or resistance.

You're able to feel a weak but definite digital pulse in the involved feet, and the hooves are slightly warm to the touch. If you're unsure, it might help to compare the heat and digital pulse of your horse's feet to those of another, unaffected horse.

Moderate founder
GRADE II

He's reluctant to move, and when you try to pick up a foot he allows it only after vigorous resistance because the added weight on the other feet magnifies his pain. When you do pick up a foot, however, you notice that he resents it when you put pressure on the sole in the toe area. This is much easier to appreciate if you use hoof testers (see *Figure 5.2*).

When standing at rest, he tends to bear more weight than usual on the hindquarters, rocking back on his haunches with his front feet held farther forward than usual, as though trying to spare his toes. His attitude is depressed, and his appetite is definitely decreased.

You're able to feel a steady, consistent digital pulse in the involved feet, and the hooves are definitely warm to the touch — there's no need to compare with a normal horse this time.

Severe founder
GRADE III

He absolutely refuses to move, and he may even be lying down. If he's down, he won't get up unless you force him to. He's deeply depressed, refuses to eat, and is totally focused on his pain. His heart and respiratory rates are elevated (over 50 beats, over 20 breaths per minute, respectively). The digital pulse is strong and obvious even to someone who ordinarily doesn't know where to find it, and the feet are literally hot to the touch. Hoof testers aren't needed to demonstrate that his toes are sore — just press on his soles at the toe with your fingers, and you'll get a painful response.

Is he ruined?

It's too soon to be thinking along these lines. Right now, at the cusp of the emergency, out there on your own, you need to do some preliminary, aggressive, no-holds-barred treatments, and you need to do them immediately because the condition can get past you in a hurry.

Later, after the first 24 hours have passed and you've had a chance to see how the horse has responded to those first treatment efforts, you can make an informed decision about whether you want to get more deeply invested. By that time, you and your horse will have managed to place yourselves securely into the hands of a competent equine veterinarian, and you can take full advantage of that vet's input, including the x-rays he/she has taken, plus your important observations of your horse's response to your initial treatments.

Nevertheless, your question is a fair one, and, for what they're worth, here are some rules of thumb regarding a founder's chances of survival:

RULE OF THUMB #1:

The worse he looks, the worse he is, but don't let that discourage you from giving your horse a fair chance.

As the grade of lameness goes up, the likelihood of permanent damage and poor prognosis also goes up — some cases are so bad that it doesn't matter how fast and hard you hit them with treatment — they're down the tubes no matter what you do. But these are the cases that were probably ongoing, subtly, for a day or two before they were noticed. Early detection and prompt, proper treatment can turn even severe cases around and leave virtually no residual damage. With your horse, the important thing to remember is that the initial treatment course is always worth a try — severe pain does not necessarily indicate that permanent damage has occurred inside the feet.

RULE OF THUMB #2:

Permanent damage is more likely if all 4 feet are involved.

When all four feet are involved, the underlying problem is a primary bodywide, septic, endotoxemic, or metabolic condition, which generally means that the cascade of destructive events going on inside his foot is going to happen faster than if only one or two feet were involved.

RULE OF THUMB #3:

Bulk is bad.

If, on top of everything else, your horse is obese for his body frame, or if he's just a big horse weighing 1200 lb or more, the odds of permanent damage (coffin bone rotation and sinking) are much increased.

RULE OF THUMB #4:

You've got 24 hours.

Most of the devastating internal damage to the laminae of the foot occurs within 24 hours of onset, so early aggressive therapy is essential even when the diagnosis is tentative.

Roughly 20% of serious founder cases won't recover satisfactorily because the underlying cause of their condition was never resolved. Statistically, 80% of all horses with severe founder have a very good chance of recovery if they're treated promptly and aggressively, even if there have already been some structural changes inside their feet.

What's going on inside?

Look at *Figures 5.1 and 5.3*. Look, specifically, at the position of the coffin bone in *Figure 5.1*: notice that the front surface of its triangular shape is exactly parallel to the front wall of the hoof. In the normal foot, it's held in that position by a delicate but firm attachment of the bone to the hoof by soft, living, gill-like interdigitating tissue called *laminae*.

At the risk of offending the designer of this system, it's a founder asking to happen. The normal blood flow to these laminae is what keeps them alive and what keeps the attachment of the bone to the hoof healthy and secure. Trouble is, that blood flow, way down there at the bottom of the foot, a good 36 inches or more below the heart, must go against gravity, from down to up, because after making the journey down the leg, the blood goes *under* the foot and then makes a U-turn. Any mishap in blood flow, any glitch in blood pressure, anything that stands in the way of that vital, nourishing blood traveling uphill through those tiny capillaries, puts the health of the laminae at serious risk.

And it doesn't take much: it can start from an innocent little reflex constriction of the blood vessels as a result of some pain or injury, or a tiny little blood clot on the loose, or a little swelling inside the foot putting extra pressure on the blood vessels — the inside of the horse's foot simply does not forgive errors. Whenever *anything* goes wrong inside the foot, founder is a real possibility.

To make matters worse, a number of chemical imbalances in some *distant* part of the body can cause those tiny capillaries in the foot to constrict, thereby pinching the already marginal blood flow and threatening the health of the laminae. And here's the clincher: if the flow of blood through those tiny capillaries is restricted even a little bit, an unfortunate bit of engineering in the foot throws a little switch and allows the blood to bypass the capillaries and take an easier detour, *around* the laminae. Now they've got no chance of getting the blood they need. Now the laminae really are in trouble.

What you see from the outside at this point is the increased digital pulse — your fingers are feeling the extra blood backing up from excessive pressure as it courses through the detour, where it does the foot absolutely no good at all. The harder that digital pulse bounces against your fingertips, the more blood is being detoured away from the laminae, and the more strangled they are — they're literally dying in there.

Meanwhile, the increased pressure in the capillaries is causing the liquid portion

FIGURE 5.1

Contrary to what was long believed, the blood supply to the laminae of the feet comes not from the coronary band above, but from a tangled bed of blood vessels below. This means that in order to nourish the vital laminae, the blood must travel against gravity, against the pressure of the horse's weight, against what often amounts to insurmountable odds.

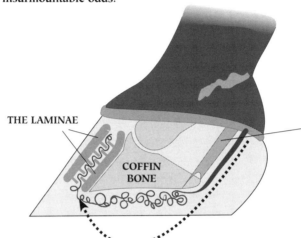

THE LAMINAE

COFFIN BONE

Normally, the deep digital flexor tendon pulls firmly on the coffin bone. If the laminae break down, there will be nothing to hold the bone in place, and the tendon will pull it away from its normal position. I.e., the bone will rotate.

FIGURE 5.2

In the early stages, hoof testers over the toe region reveal tenderness. As the case progresses, a simple pinch of the toe with bare fingers can elicit the same response.

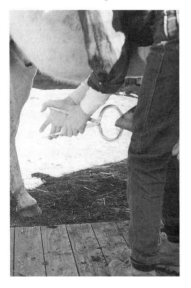

of the blood (the plasma) to leak out into the free spaces in the foot, which just makes things even tighter in there, causes even more pressure on all the blood vessels, and sets the stage for infection.

At first, the laminae are sick but still alive — they're gasping for breath, they're being strangled, but *they're not dead yet*. But with each passing minute, laminar tissue continues to degenerate and begins to die. As it dies, the delicate interdigitation of its grip that firmly held the coffin bone in position begins to loosen. Now, it's just a matter of a few shifts in the leg's position, a few tugs on the deep digital flexor tendon, before the coffin bone begins to rip away from its normal position and its tip begins to swing, or rotate, downward toward the ground. This is the beginning of the end of the foot's normal architecture. As the coffin bone rotates, the weight of the horse begins to drive the bone down toward the ground. This is called *sinking*. As a general rule, once the horse becomes a "sinker," he's a goner.

From the outside, a sinker has a concave gap just above the hoof wall (see *Figure 5.5*). The sinking and rotation further compromise blood flow because they cause tearing of more blood vessels and because the shifting weight compresses blood vessels between the ground and the sinking coffin bone. The worse it gets, the worse it gets.

FIGURE 5.3

As the coffin bone pulls away from the dying laminae that can no longer hold it in place, the deep digital flexor tendon pulls the bone even further out of position. By raising the heel 12° to 16° with a makeshift wedge, you can relax the tendon and keep it from pulling on the coffin bone.

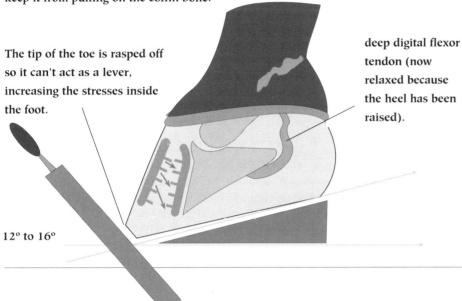

The tip of the toe is rasped off so it can't act as a lever, increasing the stresses inside the foot.

deep digital flexor tendon (now relaxed because the heel has been raised).

12° to 16°

If you think your horse may have gotten into the grain...

The initial effect of carbohydrate overload is constriction of the capillaries in the foot, which causes increased capillary pressure and movement of fluid into the open spaces inside the foot — a lot of circulatory destruction is going on, and there's not even any evidence of it on the outside. About sixteen hours after he ate the grain, the horse's heart rate increases. Mild signs of lameness begin to appear a few hours later, and within the next 24 hours that lameness develops into full-blown, severe founder — a full 40 hours *after* he ate the grain.

So if you know your horse got into the grain, don't be lulled into thinking he's okay just because he's not showing any signs of digestive upset — there's trouble brewing in his feet, and by the time that trouble is obvious, vital structures inside his feet will already have been strangled to death.

What would the vet do?

The vet would immediately try to stop the destructive cascade of events taking place inside the horse's hoof while simultaneously gathering information about how

FIGURE 5.4

The pulse at the digital artery becomes stronger, or "bounding," as the acute case of founder progresses.

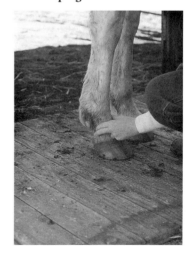

FIGURE 5.5

This horse's coffin bone has already sunken, as evidenced by the gap behind the coronary band. (Courtesy of Dr. Thomas Goetz, University of Illinois, and Veterinary Clinics of North America: Equine Practice — Vol 7, No. 1, April 1991)

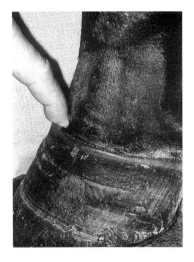

FIGURE 5.6

The surface temperature of the acutely foundering foot increases palpably as the condition progresses.

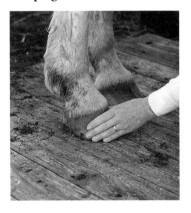

much damage has already occurred so that you could be given a reasonably accurate prediction of what the horse is going to need and what his chances are of full recovery. If you were able to provide information about what caused the founder, so much the better, because the vet could take steps to correct that problem as well. So the veterinary task is threefold:

1. Identifying and correcting the underlying problem

- If an underlying illness is suspected, diagnostic tests will be run to try and discover the cause. Possibilities include hypothyroidism, selenium deficiency, endotoxemia, kidney disease, liver disease, and infection with *Salmonella* or Potomac Horse Fever.

- If there's any possibility that the problem started in the digestive tract, mineral oil will be given by stomach tube: a gallon every two hours for one to three treatments, to block the uptake of endotoxins and to encourage whatever's in there to come out quickly, before it can be absorbed.

- If there's any possibility that the problem relates to endotoxin absorption from the gut, hyperimmune endotoxin antiserum can be given intravenously. This is a frozen plasma product, costing about $200-$300, that is the equivalent of an antidote — it's as close as you can get to a cure for endotoxemia.

- Intravenous fluids and antibiotics might be warranted, depending on what the underlying cause is suspected to be.

2. Halting the destruction inside the foot

- Immediate confinement to a small stall with clean, soft, malleable bedding such as sawdust or sand will encourage the horse to lie down.

- Immediate dietary restrictions are imposed: grass hay and room-temperature water — no grain. Bran mashes and other high-fiber, low-carbohydrate, laxative feeds might be added. If the horse is obese, his diet is further restricted.

- Pain-killing antiinflammatory drugs are given: phenylbutazone (bute), and flunixin meglumine (Banamine™). The pain causes reflex constriction of the capillaries inside the foot, which further causes strangulation of the laminae, and the pain-killing medications help to block that constrictive response. The Banamine™ has the added benefit of having some protective action against endotoxins. The potential risk of encouraging the horse to move too much, now that the pain has been reduced, is prevented by the confinement of the horse to the small stall.

- Medication is given that will encourage the circulation inside the foot to return to normal: aspirin and possibly heparin (to help dissolve and prevent the formation of blood clots — see *Special Note 5.3*), acepromazine and isoxsuprine (to dilate the constricted blood vessels), and DMSO (dimethylsulfoxide, to reduce inflammation and help the body kick out toxic chemicals trapped in the foot).

- The shoes are pulled and the feet are trimmed to shorten the toe and raise the heel, thereby helping to keep the coffin bone and hoof wall in proper alignment.

3. Formulating a prediction of expense and outcome

- X-rays are taken for baseline reference and repeated at intervals to determine whether the coffin bone is rotating and sinking.

There's no vet. What should you do?

If there's anything good about founder, this is it: Despite a lot of sophisticated research and resultant new understanding of the pathophysiology of what's happening inside the foundering foot, what to do about it when it happens as an emergency is still relatively simple and easy to do. That's good news for you, stranded without immediate veterinary service, because that means that you can take effective action right now, and as a result of that action, your horse will have a much better chance of emerging from the crisis in functional condition than if you did nothing while waiting for help.

But the action you take must be appropriate, and you must not delay, because the longer the horse goes untreated the closer he gets to the point beyond which he won't return in his former good condition. Twenty-four hours: that's your time frame — and the sooner, the better, because as you must realize by now, the problem was present before you noticed the symptoms from the outside.

Emergency treatment is a combination of medical management and therapeutic trimming to help prevent the mechanical forces that will try to wrench the coffin bone out of position. You'll try to resolve the inciting cause, minimize pain, improve the circulation inside the foot to save the beleaguered laminae, and prevent further damage. Ready? Here we go:

Confine the horse to a small area with soft bedding and enough room to lie down.

Restrict his feed to free-choice water and good quality grass hay, either ad lib (if he's not obese), or controlled amounts (if he's obese). Even if he's too thin, *do not give grain* to encourage weight gain. Ask your vet for safe, carbohydrate-free ways to bolster a founder victim's body weight.

Run cold water on the feet, or apply cold-pack wraps, to pull out the fever in the feet. If using a cold-pack wrap, replace it as soon as it loses its coolness so that the wrap doesn't hold the foot's heat *in*.

SPECIAL NOTE 5.3

Research has shown that many treatments can help after founder has started, but the only treatment that *prevented* founder in a group of horses that had an intestinal infection called DPJ (duodenitis-proximal jejunitis) was IV heparin, a "blood thinner" that keeps the blood from forming clots in the tiny blood vessels in the foot. Of 116 horses treated for DPJ, 12 were treated with heparin (none of them foundered) and 104 got all the other "usual" treatments but no heparin (31 of them foundered). You can't give heparin, but you can give another kind of "blood thinner:" *aspirin!* See the treatment section for more.

STEP 1. Confine

STEP 2.
Restrict the diet

STEP 3.
Chill

STEP 4.
Give antiinflammatories

If your regular veterinarian entrusted you with a prescription of these items, give an intramuscular injection of Banamine™ and a dose of oral bute paste or gel. See *Special Note 5.4 and 5.6* for dose recommendations.

STEP 5.
Purge

If the horse got into the grain, you'll have to try and protect him against absorbing it by encouraging as much as possible to pass through his system unabsorbed. Don't try to do this by giving mineral oil via stomach tube — the potential hazards far outweigh the potential benefits when you're not qualified to do the procedure. And force-feeding enough mineral oil orally to make a difference would also be foolhardy, since the risk is unacceptably high that some of the oil will go down "the wrong pipe" and cause aspiration pneumonia. Instead, do the next best thing: Give the horse a psyllium-oil-bran mash (see *Chapter 3* for recipe). Give two mashes, 1 hour apart, to encourage his system to empty out.

STEP 6.
Thin the blood

Give aspirin paste or gel orally, to help prevent or dissolve any blood clots in the capillaries. See *Special Note 5.5* for dose recommendations.

STEP 7.
Improve the circulation

To dilate constricted blood vessels in the foot, give an intramuscular injection of acepromazine. See *Special Note 5.7* for dose recommendations.

STEP 8.
Pull the shoes

If you know how and you have the tools, pull the shoes. If the horse absolutely can't tolerate having his foot held up for this procedure, and/or if you're not sure you can do it without damaging the hoof, skip this procedure and do step #9 *over* the shoes. If you *can* get the shoes off, then before you go on to step #9, snub the toe by rasping straight across, and round the resultant edges.

STEP 9.
Raise the heels
(yes, this is the opposite of
what was recommended
years ago...)

Apply wedges to raise the heel of both front feet (even if only one is involved) and the back feet too, if they're involved. This reduces the ability of the deep digital flexor tendon to tug the coffin bone out of position. The ideal is to raise the heel by about 12 to 16 degrees above its former position. If you don't happen to have a protractor with you to measure the angles, figure on raising the heels by about an inch — the height of a standard rubber door stop. (And, by the way, rubber doorstops make excellent emergency heel elevators — three or four per foot, depending on the size of the foot, are just the ticket.) Leave the wedges in place until you get to the vet's; the vet will decide how long to leave them on. See *Figure 5.7*.

STEP 10.
Make tracks!

Absolutely get to the vet's well within 24 hours of onset. Pull the horse trailer as close to the horse's enclosure as possible so he won't have to take any extra steps that might do more internal damage.

Things you absolutely shouldn't do, no matter who tells you to do them:

1. Some people advocate wadding up a couple rolls of gauze and taping them to the bottom of the feet to "put some pressure on the frog." They say this will keep the coffin bone from rotating. In some cases, this is a good thing to do. But if you pad or otherwise apply compression to the feet, and that compression isn't applied *exactly correctly* and sinking and/or rotation have already begun, you can actually compress the already compromised blood vessels in the sole of the foot and hasten the strangulation of the tissues inside. So, raise the heels? Yes. Apply pressure to the frog? Absolutely not. Leave this to the experts.

NO!!!
Do Not Apply Frog Pads

2. A lot of old-timers, and even a few respected books, advocate forced exercise, walking the foundering horse, as though you could "walk him out of it." Some say you should walk him on sand, because the sand will press up on his soles and keep the coffin bone from rotating. Others say that by walking the horse you're encour-aging circulation in the foot. Sounds good, right? Trouble is, walking a foundered horse is like driving a car on a flat tire — no matter what kind of surface you're traveling on, every step does more damage. Moving the foundering horse risks further ripping of the coffin bone away from its rightful position, and the more it rotates, the greater is the risk that the coffin bone will sink down toward the ground. So don't walk an acutely foundered horse — don't walk him on sand, gravel, grass, in a creek — don't walk him at all, until a good veterinarian has had a chance to assess the integrity of the foot's internal structures.

NO!!!
Do Not Walk the Horse

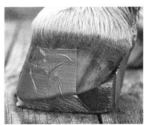

FIGURE 5.7

The heel wedge

3. Some experienced trainers know how to do nerve blocks, and you may encounter one that wants to do a nerve block on your horse's feet, to relieve the pain. *Do not allow this.* It will encourage the horse to bear weight on the foot while the circulatory difficulties are still in full force, thereby increasing the odds that the flexor tendon will rip the coffin bone away from its laminar attachment.

NO!!!
Do Not Nerve-Block the Horse

4. It may seem logical that a foundered horse's feet should be bandaged, because the soft, cushy bandage might somehow relieve the pressure on the feet. It seems logical, until you think about it: the problem is on the inside of the foot, within the rigid walls and the stiff sole. A big, padded bandage on the foot does only one positive thing: it makes *you* feel better. But what it does for the horse is mostly bad: it insulates the foot, and encourages it to hold in heat. It's akin to applying butter to a burn. So don't wrap the feet — you want to cool them, not keep them warm.

NO!!!
Do Not Bandage the Feet

One last thing to think about:

In the future, you might be able to help protect your horse against founder if he's ever stricken with an illness that causes endotoxemia. Consider vaccinating him annually with an anti-endotoxemia vaccine. Ask your veterinarian.

Why raise the heels? We used to lower them, because it seemed wise to "help the horse get off his toes" where all the pain was. But now we understand that the lower the heels are, the tighter is the pull of the deep digital flexor tendon, and it's that tendon's pull that rips the coffin bone away from its laminar attachment.

SPECIAL NOTE 5.4

BANAMINE DOSAGE FOR FOUNDER

800 lb horse:	3 cc
900 lb horse:	3-1/2 cc
1,000 lb horse:	4 cc
1,100 lb horse:	4 cc
1,200 lb horse:	4-1/2 cc
1,300 lb horse:	4-1/2 cc
1,400 lb horse:	5 cc

To be given intramuscularly, once only.

SPECIAL NOTE 5.5

ASPIRIN DOSAGE FOR FOUNDER

800 lb horse:	3 grams
900 lb horse:	4 grams
1,000 lb horse:	4-1/2 grams
1,100 lb horse:	5 grams
1,200 lb horse:	5-1/2 grams
1,300 lb horse:	6 grams
1,400 lb horse:	6-1/2 grams

To be given orally, once only.

SPECIAL NOTE 5.6

PHENYLBUTAZONE DOSAGE FOR FOUNDER

800 lb horse:	1 gram
900 lb horse:	1 gram
1,000 lb horse:	1 gram
1,100 lb horse:	1-1/2 gram
1,200 lb horse:	1-1/2 gram
1,300 lb horse:	2 grams
1,400 lb horse:	2 grams

To be given orally, once only.

SPECIAL NOTE 5.7

ACEPROMAZINE DOSAGE FOR FOUNDER

800 lb horse:	32 mg (=3.2 cc)
900 lb horse:	36 mg (=3.6 cc)
1,000 lb horse:	40 mg (=4 cc)
1,100 lb horse:	44 mg (=4.4 cc)
1,200 lb horse:	48 mg (=4.8 cc)
1,300 lb horse:	52 mg (=5.2 cc)
1,400 lb horse:	56 mg (=5.6 cc)

To be given intramuscularly, once only.

CHAPTER 6

Sudden, Severe Lamenesses

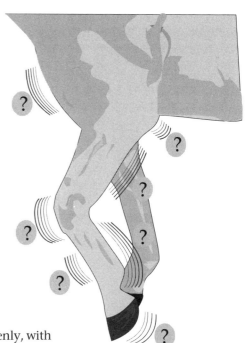

I n this chapter, we'll deal with the severe lameness that appears suddenly, with no warning, due to a traumatic injury rather than, say, illness or local infection or long-standing arthritis. Conditions that cause a gradual buildup of lameness really aren't sudden emergencies, and the gradual increase in symptoms gives you plenty of time to notice that there's a problem and summon a veterinarian — there's really no excuse for being without veterinary help in such situations. This chapter will address the most common cases of true emergency lameness, where the lameness is dramatic and severe, the symptoms appear suddenly and are often linked to an identifiable incident such as a fall or misstep or kick.

Job one: localize the problem

Your first task is to identify what area of the leg has been injured. You don't necessarily need to diagnose *what* the problem is, nor would you be expected to do so, but at the very least you need to know roughly *where* it is—whether it's hoof, lower leg, or upper leg, so that you'll know where to focus your attention.

And beware: it's easy to be misled even if you're very experienced. In fact, in some ways experience can work against you — you're so *sure* you recognize the problem that you fail to look more closely. For example, many a bowed tendon suffered critical delays in treatment because somebody misdiagnosed the problem as an abscess in the sole of the foot (a sole abscess near the heel of the sole, for example, can cause the same sort of lameness as a "fresh" bowed tendon). Learn to rely on all available clues, including your hands-on observations, and resist the temptation to make an "across the fence" diagnosis.

The sudden lamenesses most common in performance horses are discussed in this chapter. They include:

- *Puncture wounds of the hoof*
- *Bowed tendon*
- *Bucked shins/shin splints*
- *"Popped knee"*
- *Splint bone injury*
- *Tibial stress fracture*
- *Grabbed quarter*

SPECIAL NOTE 6.1

No person, no matter how big or strong, can overpower a horse. Horses employ their physical power to exercise what their instincts tell them to do in painful, scary situations: RUN! But watch a group of horses in pasture when something "alarming" happens — if the herd leader notices the "monster," assesses it, then dismisses it as non-threatening, the other members of the herd return to their grazing. They run, however, if the leader either fails to show that he's noticed and dismissed it, or if he checks it out and decides it's a threat. The experienced horseman uses this knowledge of horse nature to convince an injured horse to stop resisting treatment. Like a dominant herd leader, glare at the horse right in the eyes and give his halter a firm shake. Be serious, firm, and confident, rather than panicky and shrill, and your horse will feel less compulsion to run. Eye contact is a universal signal of dominance. Whenever possible, re-establish that eye contact to refresh your leadership and control in the situation.

What if you can't figure it out? Not to worry. With the information in this chapter, you can take steps to protect the horse against a wide range of problems. Remember, your goal is not to "cure" him, which would require a specific diagnosis. Rather, your goal is to minimize his suffering, stop the destructive cascade of events that worsen the damage after an injury has occurred, and get him the help he needs without adding to his problems.

Stop all activity.

Don't let the horse continue to hobble around in the hope that he'll "walk out of it." The decision to move the horse should be made only after you've figured out where the problem is and you've done the best you can to protect the leg against further damage.

Restraint

This is pretty basic stuff for experienced horsepeople, but for safety's sake it bears repeating. Ideally, while you're working on your horse, he'll be restrained by a trusted assistant at his head. If you're working on a hind limb, the assistant should stand on the same side, ready to pull the horse's head toward himself and lever the hindquarters away from you if problems arise. If you're working on a forelimb, the assistant should stand on the opposite side, ready to pull the forequarters toward himself, away from you. Physical restraint devices, such as a twitch, lip chain or rope, chin chain or rope, war bridle, etc., can be both potentially helpful and potentially dangerous, depending on the horse and on your own experience in using them — use these tools only if you're well versed in their proper use and you're familiar with the horse's response to them. In the majority of cases, a thoughtful, cautious, horseman's approach is a safer policy than exceptional restraint measures.

If it's necessary to tie the horse, don't cross-tie him — he can rear and lunge forward when in cross-ties. And avoid close quarters so you can get out of harm's way should the horse lash out in pain or fall or otherwise make a sudden change in position. *Never* attempt to examine an injured horse in a standing tie-stall or in a horse trailer.

No drugs.

The use of chemical restraint — tranquilizers, sedatives and pain killers— is unwise in the field lameness situation. Such drugs can mask the symptoms, making your detective work more difficult, and they can also affect the horse's balance, making it less likely that he will be able to stand during your examination without risk of stumbling or falling — in addition to being hazardous to your health, additional damage can occur to an already injured leg if the horse feels the need to suddenly bear weight on the limb to "catch himself." Furthermore, when under the influence of a mood-altering sedative or tranquilizer, some horses seem oblivious to painful stimuli but can suddenly overreact in an excessive and illogical manner when you least expect it. Besides, the tranquilizing effects are easily overridden when pain registers, and some tranquilized horses actually seem more agitated than before the drug was given. You don't need any more surprises right now.

Start your examination.

Start at the hoof and work your way up. First, examine the outside of the hoof wall and coronary band in its natural position, then lift the foot (see *Special Note 6.2*) and examine the sole thoroughly, including the frog, its central cleft, and the sulci. Look for cuts, spots of blood, discolorations, or something "obvious" (and often missed) such as a a nail. Be gentle and on guard for sudden reactions if you happen to touch or shift the injured area inadvertently. If you do get such a reaction, make full use of it — it's a valuable clue.

Slowly and methodically work your way up the leg, inspecting each area visually first, then with gentle fingertips, followed by a moderate pressing or squeezing with your fingers to see if you can feel excess heat, any spongy swellings, a crackly, bubbly feeling in the tissues called *crepitus*, and to see if you can elicit a pain reaction. Finally, as you encounter each joint, gently put it through its normal range of motion: side-to-side, front-to-back, joystick, then rotation or "door-knob" movement. Look, touch, gently press and squeeze, and "work" the joints, in that order, all the way up the horse's leg, while watching for painful reactions. And remember that there can be more than one injury.

Heat and swelling can be valuable sign-posts directing you to where the injury is. But if the injury just happened, you might find no abnormal heat, little if any swelling, and no bounding pulse (throbbing). Why? Because the injury just happened. All injuries cause inflammation — it's a necessary component of the healing process, bringing increased circulation to the area to support new tissue growth and facilitate the removal of dead tissue and other debris — and inflammation has three main "side-effects": heat, swelling, and pain. But if this injury just happened, there hasn't been time for billboard-type inflammation to develop, so it might be more difficult to localize the problem — you might have to rely entirely on your other clues (what you saw happen, how the horse is holding or using the leg, your ability to identify crepitus, and/or your ability to elicit and recognize a painful response from the horse).

If you're successful in locating the injury this early in the game, before inflammation sets in, there's a very big payoff: your treatment at this early stage will be more effective, secondary damage will be halted or minimized, and the prognosis for future use is maximized. If the injury happened more than fifteen minutes ago,

SPECIAL NOTE 6.2

Pay close attention to the clues your horse gives you. If he reacts in pain when you pick up his foot, note the reaction and put it back down — his injury might involve a joint, or there might be a fracture, or the extensor tendons at the front of the leg might be damaged, all of which would make flexing the leg excruciating.

In almost every injury, the damage done to the tissues by the initial insult is doubled by inflammation after the injury — unless you know what to do, and you do it FAST. Don't waste time. With every passing minute, the damaged area spreads, threatening to leave a bigger scar and potentially permanent disability.

inflammation has already begun to develop, and the specific damaged area may be swollen and warm. This can make the injury easier to locate, but the longer the delay, the more catching up you'll have to do in the area of treatment.

Once you've located the injury, your attention will focus on preventing further damage, damage that will result either from harmful movements by the horse, or from out-of-control inflammation. It's true that inflammation is "a necessary component of the healing process," but in almost every injury, in almost every species including human, the damage done to the tissues by the initial insult is *doubled* by the secondary damage from inflammation. Why? Because in most cases inflammation goes overboard — it is more severe than it "needs" to be — and it causes excessive pressure, hinders drainage, and interferes with circulation, all of which can expand the area of damage, prolong healing time, and increase the chance that excess scar tissue, disfigurement, and decreased function will result. So don't waste time. With every passing minute, the damage and the prognosis worsen.

THE FOOT

Puncture wounds of the foot

It's hard to find a barnyard, particularly on an older farmstead, that doesn't have bolts and nails "growing" out of the ground, and penetrating hoof wounds are, as a result, very common. Most occur when the horse is free in an area where such "pokers" persist, despite vigilant efforts to remove them from the premisis, or a former construction site where discarded welding rods, shards of glass, scraps of metal and sharp wedges of wood are present, or where brush and small trees have been cleared and short, small-diameter stumpage has been left firmly rooted into the ground, ready to penetrate a passing hoof. Fallen or pruned branches of thorn-bearing bushes are another common source of penetrating hoof wounds.

Often, once the "poker" has been removed, there's little or no pain — it isn't the nail (or whatever) that really hurts — it's the inflammation and pressure that develop later. That's one of the dangerous things about puncture wounds — if the horse isn't dramatically lame, his injury might not get the attention it deserves until infection is rampant.

How do you identify a penetrating hoof wound?

If you're lucky, the wound has just occurred and the foreign body (let's call it a "poker") is still in place in the horse's hoof. In most cases, even if the poker penetrated vital structures inside the hoof, the level of pain is markedly reduced the minute the poker is removed. In that case, identifying a penetrating hoof wound may depend on pure luck — you saw it happen, or just happened to find the entry hole when cleaning the hoof. Otherwise, you might be unaware of the injury until the resultant infection has caused a gradual return of the pain — in that situation, you will have had time to notice the problem and get help, but you should also know that the necessary delay in getting that help has already put your horse's future in a precarious position. So let's limit this discussion to the acute emergency — you've just discovered that the puncture has occurred.

What's going on inside the foot as a result of the injury?

The big question is, did the poker penetrate vital structures, such as a joint, or a tendon, or bone, or the navicular bursa — or — did it miss vital structures and penetrate only the digital cushion (see *Figure 6.2*)? The answer depends on:

√   where the poker entered the foot (the "toe zone," the "central zone or the "heel zone"),
√   the angle it went in, and
√   how deep it went.

FIGURE 6.1

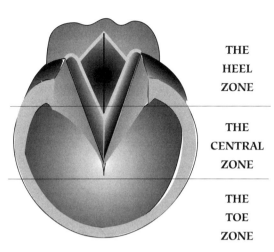

THE HEEL ZONE

THE CENTRAL ZONE

THE TOE ZONE

By far, the most dangerous place for a deep, penetrating hoof wound is the central zone, because so many vital structures lie within it.

If vital structures were missed, the resulting infection will be relatively trivial in its consequences, and your horse will probably be okay with proper treatment. But if vital structures were invaded by the poker, your horse may be in serious trouble, and the ultimate outcome may be loss of function, loss of career, maybe even loss of life.

Let's be realistic

University veterinarians, who see only the cases that didn't go well under the care of the field vet, might be surprised to know how often horses step on nails or other pokers and emerge unscathed. It's remarkable, the number of penetrating hoof wounds that result in a temporary, trivial lameness that responds beautifully to a few shots of penicillin, or a week or two of ostrich-style neglect. That's the good news — the odds are with you, especially if the poker penetrated no deeper than about half an inch.

But you'd shudder if you knew how devastating a penetrating hoof wound can be — university veterinarians see these devastating cases all the time, and they're an awful mess. Horses that are perfectly healthy otherwise... euthanized because the nail they stepped on penetrated something important within the foot, and it was badly contaminated, and it didn't get treated vigorously from the start, and now, months later, they're three-legged lame with a chronic, draining, rotten infection deep within the tissues of the foot. Once the fire is started inside the hoof, it's very, very difficult to put it out, and while it burns it does permanent damage to joints, tendons, bone and cartilage. Can you afford to hide your head in the sand and take your chances, or is it worth it to assume the worst when your horse gets a penetrating hoof wound and practice a little preventive medicine? It's up to you.

Why is this injury dangerous?

You can only guess where the tip of poker reached inside the hoof. To make an educated guess, divide the bottom of the hoof into the three zones and look at what structures are in harm's way (see *Figure 6.1 and 6.2*).

The common, ominous thread binding all puncture wounds is that the longer the interval of time between the initial injury and treatment, the higher the potential for serious consequences. An established infection within the structures of the hoof rarely resolves with conservative treatment (soaking the foot, infusing antiseptics into the puncture wound, and giving systemic antibiotics) — major surgery is almost always required, and it's not always successful. At this moment, your horse's freshly wounded hoof is not infected — it's just contaminated. Quick action might be able to prevent infection.

What would the vet do?

If the poker were metal, the vet would take x-rays of the hoof before removing it in order to see which, if any, vital structures might lie in its path. Then he/she would anesthetize the horse, trim and scrub the hoof, remove the poker, and with sterile, sharp instruments, enlarge the entry hole and remove any debris introduced by the poker. If the poker broke off a piece of the coffin bone, the piece would be removed at this time, as would any other tissues of the foot that appear to have been contaminated.

Next, the vet would irrigate the tract left by the poker, first using sterile saline (salt) solution, and possibly ending with an antiseptic solution such as 1% povidone iodine (Betadine®) to kill bacteria and fungi. Since most puncture wounds are contaminated with a "potpourri" of bacteria, antiseptic solutions are generally preferred over antibiotics — antibiotics are usually reserved for situations where a particular bug is the target. Regardless of the choice of flushing solutions, the vet should be careful to infuse them into the hole with only enough pressure to flush it out — if excessive pressure is used to infuse the flushing solution, debris and bacteria might be forced deeper into tissues that heretofore were uncontaminated, thus making the situation worse.

However, one particular bacterium is especially problematic in puncture wounds of the foot: it's called *Clostridium tetani* — the bug that causes tetanus. In addition to keeping the horse up-to-date on his tetanus vaccinations, there are three direct ways to prevent tetanus bacteria from setting up housekeeping in a wound:

1. Reduce the *number* of bacteria present by physically removing as much of the wound's contamination and bacteria as possible in the initial cleaning and debridement. That is, make the entire extent of the wounded area as clean as possible, by removing the tiniest particles of contaminating material, and by removing any

FIGURE 6.2

THE TOE ZONE

A poker penetrating the toe zone can strike the coffin bone, risking infection (osteomyelitis), possibly even a fracture. Unlike the long, hard bones of the leg, the coffin bone is rather delicate, shaped like a wedge of pumice stone with brittle edges that can break off.

Once an infection is established in the bone, surgery will be needed to remove all questionable tissue, *plus* a long, intense course of expensive antibiotics, *plus* incredibly good luck. At best, it's a salvage procedure — the odds of the horse returning to pre-injury performance levels are slim unless it's detected and caught early, before the bone is invaded by infection.

THE CENTRAL ZONE

The central zone is packed with vulnerable structures, including the coffin bone (risk: osteomyelitis), and the coffin *joint* (risk: septic arthritis). If the joint becomes infected, permanent lameness can result. At the time of the injury, what you have is a *contaminated* joint. Within hours, it'll be *infected*.

Other important targets in the central zone include the superficial digital flexor tendon (risk: septic tenosynovitis), the navicular bursa (risk: septic bursitis), and the navicular bone (risk: more osteomyelitis).

STRUCTURES AT RISK:

a. coffin bone
b. coffin joint
c. deep digital flexor tendon and its sheath
d. navicular bone
e. navicular bursa (a "cushion" between the navicular bone and the tendon)
f. lateral cartilages
g. digital cushion

THE HEEL ZONE

The main structures to avoid in the heel zone are the lateral cartilages ("wings") of the coffin bone. Infection here can cause a condition called quittor, a chronic, smelly, soupy, draining mess that has little chance of healing without surgery because cartilage has essentially no blood supply. In order to remove all infected tissue, the surgeon has to be brutal.

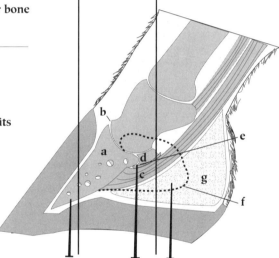

tissues that appear to be contaminated or damaged.

2. Introduce oxygen into the wound. The tetanus bugs prefer to live in an anaerobic environment — where there is no oxygen — that's why they "love" puncture wounds that get sealed over, sealing out the oxygen supply.

3. Infuse a tetanus-hating antibiotic solution into the wound and into the animal's general system. As dangerous as the tetanus bug is, most antibiotics can kill it if they can get to it.

Removing all the debris and contaminated tissue is the most important part of the treatment process — all the antiseptics and antibiotics in the world will not make up for a hit-or-miss job of physically cleaning the entire extent of the wound.

Opening or widening the wound surgically is one way of keeping the deeper recesses of the wound oxygenated, thereby discouraging tetanus from setting up housekeeping.

If the enlarged part of the hole is no deeper than 3/4 of an inch, the vet might infuse it gently with hydrogen peroxide 3% USP, which is the standard peroxide solution available for about 50ç per pint in any pharmacy. Peroxide releases oxygen as it bubbles, creating an oxygen-rich environment that tetanus bugs can't tolerate.

Before the hole has been enlarged, however, peroxide should be avoided, because the pressure created by the bubbling action can build if the narrow hole becomes clogged with foam, and that pressure can force particles of debris deeper into the foot, thus making an out-of-reach infection more likely. And if, after surgery, the hole is so deep that the flushing solution might go in and spread around instead of coming right back out again, peroxide would not be a good choice because it can be irritating. In either of these cases, the vet would be more likely to infuse a solution of penicillin, using a penicillin product designed for intravenous use (not the creamy white product used in intramuscular injections). The tetanus bug is very sensitive to good old-fashioned penicillin.

Depending on the internal structures involved in the wound, the vet might install a surgical drain into the foot — this is particularly likely if the navicular bursa or the coffin joint was contaminated by the injury. A surgical drain is nothing more than a strip of an inert material such as latex that is inserted into a contaminated area to keep it open and provide a pathway for accumulating liquids to leak out alongside the drain.

The rim of the hole is then plugged with a sterile wad of Betadine®-soaked cotton or gauze, and the entire hoof is bandaged with a waterproof dressing to keep dirt, manure, and bedding material from getting up into the hole. The horse is kept in a diligently cleaned hospital stall to further limit the potential for contamination.

The horse's tetanus vaccination status is investigated and updated if necessary. If he's had a tetanus toxoid vaccine within the past six months, a "booster" of tetanus toxoid is given; if not, the vet might give an injection of tetanus *antitoxin*, with or without a second injection containing the *toxoid* . See *Special Note 6.5)*

To help ensure that the deep structures of the foot do not develop an infection from any contamination remaining in the tract, the vet might prescribe a minimum ten-day treatment course of systemic broad-spectrum antibiotics, injectable or oral, being certain to select a product that will kill tetanus organisms if necessary.

To hold inflammation and pain at a minimum, the horse is also put on a daily schedule of an antiinflammatory like phenylbutazone ("bute") or flunixin meglumine (Banamine™) for a period of three days to two weeks, depending on the level of pain. This will help to combat inflammation and keep the area from swelling shut, and it will also relieve pain and encourage the horse to bear weight on the injured foot, thereby increasing circulation, encouraging drainage, and protecting the other three

Beware of tetanus! The horse, more than any other species, is especially vulnerable to tetanus. And wouldn't you know it — the horse lives in an environment that is virtually boiling over with tetanus organisms.

legs against breakdown from bearing too much weight.

Bandage changes, soakings, and wound irrigation with antiseptic solutions are usually done daily until the hole fills, from the inside out, with healthy, soft pink tissue — this should take about a week. It can take several weeks for harder hoof horn to cover over, and protective measures such as a hoof boot or a padded shoe might be warranted.

There's no vet. What should you do?

Restrain the horse *on a clean surface* such as concrete, fresh clean grass, or a drop cloth. Do not place the foot back down onto the ground until the surface has been swept clean to prevent further contamination from entering the hole. Clean the foot thoroughly, then pull out the poker, being careful not to break it off, pulling it in the same plane as it went in. As you're removing it, memorize where it entered, how deep it went, and in what direction it was aiming — these holes have a habit of disappearing. In fact, it's not uncommon to forget which foot was involved! Save the poker for future reference.

STEP 1.
Choose your working area and clean the foot.

Assume that *every* vital structure inside the foot has been contaminated. You will now take steps to minimize the damage done by that theoretical worst-case scenario. If you were wrong, no harm done, but if you do not act aggressively and you find out later that you should have, by then it might be too late to save your horse.

STEP 2.
Assume the worst.

With a clean, sharp, narrow-bladed, flame-sterilized hoof knife, trim away all ragged, old, and soiled edges and surfaces of hoof wall, sole, frog, and sulci to create an entirely fresh, clean surface. Leave no nook or cranny unpared — such cul-de-sacs can harbor pockets of bacteria to contaminate the wound hole and cause infection. Re-sterilize your hoof knife often.

STEP 3.
Trim the whole foot.

Pare away the edges of the entry hole at the surface of the hoof to enlarge it to at least twice its original diameter. If you stay at the surface, your knife is very sharp, and you pare away only small slivers of material with each cut, this should not be painful for the horse, and it should not cause any bleeding. If your knife becomes dull, sharpen and re-sterilize it — a dull knife requires more pressure to cut through the hoof horn, and that pressure can be painful, provoking the horse to jerk the foot away from you, risking further injury and contamination. Clean the ground surface often so that the hoof will not become re-contaminated if you have to set it down.

STEP 4.
Widen the hole.

Now it's time to work more deeply. Gradually, taking tiny little curls of hoof material with each bite and re-sterilizing your knife often, enlarge the tract made by the path of the poker, making a funnel-shaped hole that is widest at the bottom (the sole of

STEP 5.
Make a funnel.

the foot). Ignore old book advice to make the hole "dime-sized" — that's too big. All you're trying to do is pare away all surfaces that were touched by the poker, and in the process, you'll be widening the hole just enough to make sure it stays open for oxygen to go in and debris to come out. Take care to remove any debris as well as any contaminated or soiled hoof material encountered along the way. Go no deeper than 1/2", even if the poker went deeper than that, because your field environment is not surgically sterile and you risk further contamination of vital tissues with your efforts.

STEP 6.
Flush the enlarged, cleaned hole.

Once you've finished "digging," drizzle a capful of peroxide into the hole (*don't squirt it in under pressure*), quickly place a half-inch stack of sterile gauze 4 x 4 squares over the hole, tape them onto the foot to prevent dirt or other contaminating material from entering it, and let the horse set his foot down for a couple of minutes (onto the *clean* ground surface — no loose dirt or manure) to allow the peroxide and any debris, blood, or other contaminants to gravitate out the hole you've so nicely enlarged.

STEP 7.
Lather, rinse, repeat.

Pick up the foot, remove the gauze pads, and wipe away the dirty foam bubbled out by the peroxide. Rinse the hole by *drizzling* (not blasting) sterile eye wash from a squirt bottle into the hole until it overflows. No high-pressure streams, please — this can blast bacteria and debris deeper into the foot. Tape a fresh stack of sterile gauze 4 x 4 squares over the hole and set the foot down again, allowing the liquid to drain out. Then repeat this flushing procedure over and over again, first with peroxide, then with the eye wash, until no more contamination is draining from the hole — the gauze squares are moist from the wash solution, but they're not discolored or dirty. Be sure to end with a rinse cycle — don't leave peroxide in there, because it can be irritating.

STEP 8.
Disinfect.

Now drizzle the tamed-iodine antiseptic solution Betadine® or its generic equivalent (use the *solution*, not the *scrub*, which contains a detergent) into the hole until it overflows. Do not inject it under pressure with a syringe, as this may force any debris remaining in the tract farther up into vulnerable areas deeper within the foot. Be sure to use *tamed* iodine, not the "strong iodine solution" that is popular among farriers — it is extremely caustic and will burn delicate internal structures. And don't use "tincture of iodine" either — this is also too strong, and it contains alcohol, which does not belong inside the foot.

STEP 9.
Plug the hole.

Wedge a Betadine®-soaked cotton ball partially into the hole so that it can easily be pulled out with your fingers. Cover the sole with another half-inch stack of gauze 4"x4" squares soaked in Betadine® solution, and wrap the entire foot with Vetrap™ to hold the squares onto the foot.

Cover the entire Vetrap™-wrapped foot with duct tape to make the dressing somewhat waterproof and strong enough to hold together, and to keep the foot clean. Or, better yet, slip the bandaged foot into a sturdy, waterproof, clean plastic hoof boot (see *Figure 6.3*).

STEP 10.

Waterproof and dirt-proof the foot.

Take care of tetanus vaccination needs: If the horse has had a tetanus toxoid injection within the past six months, give a "booster" of tetanus toxoid intramuscularly (see *Chapter 2: Giving Shots*). If not, give tetanus antitoxin, 1500 IU, intramuscularly, and a tetanus toxoid injection in a separate spot. See *Special Note 6.5* about possible hazards of using tetanus antitoxin.

STEP 11.

TETANUS!

Give an antiinflammatory drug such as oral phenylbutazone ("bute") to minimize pain and inflammation (see *Special Note 6.3* for dose).

STEP 12.

Give an antiinflammatory.

Should you seek veterinary assistance?

It's a good idea, within 24 hours of the initial injury, unless you're *positive* that the poker penetrated less than one-half inch. In that case what you've done will probably be enough. Nevertheless, it shouldn't be difficult for you to get to a competent equine vet in 24 hours. In doing so, you'll benefit from getting a second, experienced, opinion, backed by such wonderful tools as x-rays (the vet can infuse the tract with a contrast medium such as barium and see where it leads, and he can see whether the coffin bone has been fractured), ultrasound (the vet can infuse the tract with sterile water and see how deeply the tract extends, and where it leads), anesthesia (the vet can probe and dig more deeply than you did without fear of causing pain), surgical

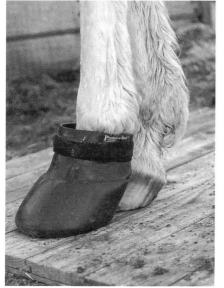

FIGURE 6.3

After meticulously cleaning the foot and carefully excavating and irrigating the puncture wound, a plastic hoof boot like this one is invaluable for preserving the clean environment you've worked so hard to create. Bandages and duct tape are fine if the horse is to be confined to a stall with soft bedding, but if he must walk any distance to get to veterinary assistance, the bandage is likely to wear through and expose the foot to dirt, mud, grit, and a whole host of willing contaminants. The boot should be water tight (the plastic models seem to hold up better than the rubber ones), tall enough to encompass the pastern, large enough to put on over the foot bandage, and somewhat contoured to the shape of the foot. It should be removed and cleaned daily along with the bandage.

instruments (they're sterile, and they're made for digging around in wounds), and specialists on the other end of the telephone (the vet can call upon experts at private practices and veterinary universities all across the globe, asking for advice if he/she encounters problems or has questions about your case). It's your call, but if I were you, I'd get to the vet. And if the horse becomes more, rather than less, sore over the next few days, take that as a sign that there's trouble brewing, and get to a veterinarian right away.

What's the prognosis?

It all depends on two things: how deep the poker went, and how long the delay between the initial injury and appropriate treatment. The deeper the wound, and the longer the delay, the worse the prognosis. If the horse's pain escalates over the course of the next few days, there's probably an infection and/or tissue death inside the foot, and you're probably in trouble.

What about follow-up care?

Twice a day, soak the foot in a strong solution of Epsom salts. Take the boot or bandage off, stuff the hole with a fresh, Betadine®-soaked cotton ball, and wrap the "naked" foot with a clean roll of gauze bandage — this will act as a "filter" to keep particles of debris from floating into the hole — and place the gauze-wrapped foot into the bucket. Stand next to the horse, keeping your hand on the bucket handle at all times. If he picks up his foot, lift the bucket up with the foot to keep it submerged and to keep the solution from spilling. Soak for ten minutes, then remove the gauze and cotton ball and pat the foot dry with a clean towel. Fill the hole with Betadine™, let it drain out, and re-bandage as before: wedged-in Betadine™-soaked cotton ball, stack of Betadine™-soaked gauze 4 x 4 squares, Vetrap™, then duct tape or plastic boot. If using the plastic boot, wash, disinfect, and dry it thoroughly before putting it back on.

Grabbed quarter

This is an injury to the soft tissue of the heel and quarter area of the front foot, usually occurring when the horse overreaches with hind shoe and grabs the quarter from the front foot. It's especially common when the horse stumbles and scrambles to catch himself.

What you see from the outside

If it's minor, a small flap of the bulb of the heel has been peeled down. If it's serious, a significant portion of the heel has been sheared away, perhaps including the coronary band.

What's going on inside

Superficial grabbed quarters are the same as any other surface abrasion: the remaining tissues are inflamed, contaminated, and bleeding from damaged small blood vessels. Deeper grabbed quarters that involve the coronary band are distinguished by the loss of tissue that is needed for continued normal growth and maintenance of hoof horn.

What would the vet do?

The treatment challenge is related to the location of the injury: it's an area that's difficult to bandage and nearly impossible to keep clean. Severe cases might require general anesthesia in order to clean and trim away damaged tissues and create a clean, raw surface for healing. The resultant wound is dressed and bandaged, and the horse is confined to a clean, straw-bedded stall with frequent bandage changes until the wound has healed.

There's no vet. What should you do?

Even though there may be a large chunk of tissue missing, and even though part of the missing tissue might include coronary band, don't panic — the foot and hoof wall can regenerate all their components, including coronary band. Your main challenge will be to get the wounded area clean and keep it clean.

Move the horse to a well-drained area and thoroughly wash the entire foot, from fetlock down, using plenty of Ivory soap and a running hose. Wash and wash until the whole foot is squeaky clean and the rinse water shows no traces of dirt.

Dip a brand new, soft, children's toothbrush in betadine scrub (the kind that sudses) and gently but vigorously scrub the raw, exposed tissues. The horse should tolerate this quite well, as the hosing will have effectively numbed the area.

Using a mild salt solution (see *Special Note 6.6*), rinse vigorously, with the foot well elevated on a draining surface so it doesn't get muddy or gritty from water splasing back up onto the foot. By this point, the wounded area should look very clean and pink, with no traces of dirt or grit visible on its surface or in any of the nooks and crannies.

If a flap of tissue has been formed, press it firmly into its proper position. If, however, tissue has been sheared completely off, have a stack of clean 4 x 4 gauze sponges ready. Blanch a section of the wound with a 1/2 inch stack of sponges — it will take about two seconds for the oozing blood to reappear — and while it's clean and dry, quickly spray that area with Nexaband™ aerosol. Continue with this dab-spray, dab-spray process until the entire wounded area is coated with the Nexaband™. Once an area

Don't panic if part of the coronary band is missing — it can regenerate.

SPECIAL NOTE 6.6

Homemade Saline Solution
Mix 1 tsp table salt per 1 quart cool, clean water.

STEP 1.
Wash the wound.

STEP 2.
Gentle surgical scrub.

STEP 3.
Final rinse.

STEP 4.
"Seal" it.
If your vet entrusted you with an emergency prescription of Nexaband™ aerosol, use it now.

is treated, do not disturb it or you'll possibly rub off the coating and start it bleeding again. (If you don't have Nexaband™, skip to Step 5).

STEP 5.
Wrap it.
Note: if you have no Nexa-band™, apply triple antibiotic first aid ointment to the stack before placing it over the wound.

Make a 1/2 inch thick stack of clean, soft gauze sponges, staggering them to make the wad wide enough to cover the entire wound, and place them over the wound, then secure the stack in place with a roll of fluffy Kling gauze, being sure to wrap around the entire foot. Now apply a roll of 2-inch wide cast padding, again covering the entire foot, and cover the whole thing with a roll of Vetrap™. Finally, to keep the bandage clean and dry, apply a layer of duct tape (See *Chapter 18*).

STEP 6.
Confine.

Keep the horse confined to a clean stall with minimal bedding. Keep the stall impeccably clean and change the bandage daily, carefully cleaning the wound before applying the new bandage. If it's gooey and/or foul smelling, the Nexaband™ seal will be ruined. But that's okay — just clean it and re-apply the bandage using triple antibiotic first aid ointment on your stack of gauze sponges, and do more frequent bandage changes to keep the tissues cleaner.

Should I seek veterinary assistance?

That shouldn't be necessary unless the wound is so deep that you think vital structures (such as the flexor tendons) might be involved — then a veterinary assessment is a very good idea. If you have any doubt, have it checked out. If it turns out that deeper structures are damaged, the vet may decide that a cast should be applied.

THE LOWER LEG

Your examination tells you that your horse's injury is in his lower leg, between the coronary band and the knee or hock joint.

Following is a description of five of the most common emergency injuries of the lower legs of performance horses, including bowed tendons, bucked shins, shin splints, splint bone injuries, and carpal joint injuries.

Read the descriptions of these conditions and find the one that most closely matches what you're seeing in your horse. Then read on for a detailed explanation of that injury's consequences, what the vet would do, and your best course of emergency treatment if veterinary assistance is not available. Remember, the goal here is to exercise damage control, to stop the cascade of destructive events that is occurring on the inside of the injured leg, and to keep the horse from injuring himself further while you get him to the trailer, loaded, and transported to a qualified equine veterinarian for x-rays and a definitive diagnosis. In nature, the injury will get much worse before it gets better. Your goal is to change nature's plan and preserve your horse's athletic future.

Bowed Tendon

This injury is a sudden tearing—partial or complete—of one or both of the two flexor tendons. It's also called tendinitis, or tendon sprain. By definition, bowed tendon always involves the SDF and/or the DDF (superficial digital flexor or deep digital flexor) tendons that run down the back of the lower legs. These tendons serve to flex the fetlocks (fore- and hind-limbs), flex the "knee" [carpus] (fore-limb) and straighten the hock (hind-limb). See *Figure 6.4*.

What are the most common causes of bowed tendon?

1. Chronic overwork and fatigue of the tendons that run down the back of the cannon bone. In most cases, this type of bowed tendon occurs in the front limbs and is most common in professional working racehorses.

2. Accident — a misstep, a fall, a slip or stumble, that places a sudden and overwhelming stress on those tendons. This type will occur with equal frequency in front or back limbs, and it's the most common type of bowed tendon injury in amateur performance and pleasure horses, particularly those on weekend-warrior work/play schedules.

3. An external blow to the tendons, such as a kick.

What you see

In mild cases or the early stages of more severe cases, the evidence can be very subtle — little or no lameness at first, only slight tenderness to finger pressure along the midsection of the tendon along the back of the cannon bone, and a slight increase in warmth in the damaged area. The horse might stand on the leg but shift weight back and forth frequently between left and right sides, holding the injured limb in partial flexion when weight is on the other leg.

This subtlety is often what leads to more damage — if the lameness were more obvious, it would attract more attention and get treatment right away. Instead, it goes unnoticed, the horse is encouraged to keep moving, more fibers are damaged, they bleed and inflame, causing edema and hemorrhage that damages even more fibers. As the swollen, ragged tendon moves with the horse's every step, it chatters against its enveloping sheath instead of gliding smoothly the way it did before the injury. The friction irritates the sheath, which swells, which makes it even tighter and increases the friction. Instead of a silver band inside a silk sheath, the tendon becomes a rapidly fraying rope.

HOW DID IT HAPPEN?

"He slipped."

"He almost fell."

"He stepped into a hole."

"He raced well, but near the end of the run, he pulled up lame."

"The arena was deep mud and slippery."

Bowed tendon is common in horses that belong to "weekend warrior" riders who hurl themselves onto soft, out-of-shape horses on weekends and ride hard, with reckless abandon, across uneven terrain.

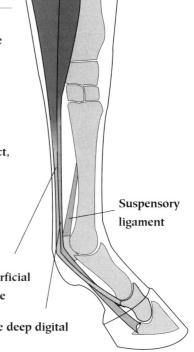

FIGURE 6.4

THE NORMAL LEG

The main tendons supporting the back of the leg are smooth, glistening, and very strong. Their superior fibers can only be made while the horse is still a fetus, still inside his mother. When those perfect fibers are injured in a performing horse, they can only be replaced by an inferior fiber that is weaker, less elastic, and instead of being organized in perfect, parallel bundles, they're arranged in a haphazard way that makes the healed tendon enlarged, lumpy, and a blaring advertisement that says, "This leg is damaged goods." Re-injury is virtually guaranteed unless the initial injury is handled properly.

Suspensory ligament

Tendon of the superficial digital flexor muscle

Tendon of the deep digital flexor muscle

In severe cases, the lameness is anything but subtle. The involved leg is held in passive partial-flexion at rest, and when on the move, the horse shows a dramatic head-bobbing lameness. Hands-on exam reveals pain in the tendon behind the cannon bone, usually at mid-cannon level if it's a typical case involving only the SDF tendon. In some cases, however, the DDF tendon is also involved, and the swelling extends lower, sometimes including the fetlock joint. As the length of time from the injury increases, and as the severity of the injury goes up the scale, there will be heat and increasing swelling over the injured area (the swelling may remain localized in the injured region, or it may spread out to involve the entire tendon, fetlock, and pastern region depending on the severity of the injury).

So: the symptoms and their magnitude will depend on the severity of the injury and the length of time between the incident and the examination.

- Lameness on the move will range from subtle hesitation or shortened stride at the trot, to severe, obvious lameness at the walk.

- In the undisturbed, at-rest state, the horse's discomfort will range from mild ("restless leg syndrome," shifting weight from leg to leg as though the affected leg aches) to severe ("three-legged horse," the affected leg is held up or rested in the slightly flexed position with the toe of the hoof touching the ground).

FIGURE 6.5

THE CLASSIC BOWED TENDON

Most bowed tendons involve only the superficial digital flexor tendon, and most of the damage occurs in the tendon's midsection. When the fibers of the tendon are stretched beyond their elastic ability, they tear, and the damaged fibers bleed. Blood leaks into the body of the tendon itself, painfully separating the fibers, furthering the damage, and hastening the onset of inflammation. As the heat, swelling, and pain magnify with each passing minute, the diagnosis becomes easier and easier to discern — it's just waiting for your fingertips.

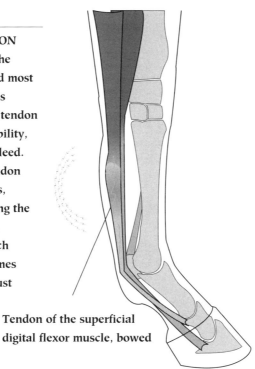

Tendon of the superficial
digital flexor muscle, bowed

- There will be swelling and heat, ranging from localized sponginess and subtle warmth over the injured area of tendon, to severe swelling and distinct heat over the entire lower leg including pastern, fetlock, and the entire cannon bone area.

- And there will be pain on finger pressure, ranging from a barely perceptible flinch to a sudden rearing and jerking away of the affected limb.

How can you be sure it's a bowed tendon?

To confirm a suspected bowed tendon, start by examining the tendon with the leg in its natural position, which will either be in the normal standing, weight-bearing position, or in the slightly flexed, resting on the toe position, depending on the severity of the horse's pain.

1. Look at the groove that normally separates the tendons from the back of the cannon bone in a normal horse, or in any of your horse's normal, unaffected legs, then compare to the affected leg: look for a filling of that groove, indicating swelling.

2. Gently feel the lateral edges of the tendon's entire length, from top (carpus or hock) to bottom (over the fetlock and down the pastern), looking for any areas where the usually distinct edges of the tendon are "muddled," or less "sharp."

Bowed tendon is common in a horse asked to perform athletic feats he's not conditioned for — his muscles aren't strong enough to bear their share of the load, so the burden is carried by the tendons. Trouble is, those tendons can tear if stretched too far. Fatigue, incoordination, deep or uneven or slippery footing, improper shoeing (long toe, low heel configuration) or long feet overdue for farriery, set the stage. When the elastic fibers of the flexor tendons are stretched beyond their normal limits, they pull apart from each other, sometimes actually tearing the entire tendon in two.

Bowed tendon is the most feared injury among horse trainers because horses with "bows" are least likely to return to full performance, and those that do are almost guaranteed to re-injure.

In an uninjured leg, the tendon should be easily identified with your fingers, and its edges should feel like a flat steel plate when the horse is bearing weight.

3. Apply gentle pressure with a slight pinching action, looking for a spongy feeling of the tendon or the sheath that surrounds it — if necessary, compare to a known-normal leg.

4. Look for a reaction of pain by applying a slightly firmer pinching action, starting at the top and working your way down — if you find a painful spot, check it again, just to make sure. Remember, injury to the outermost, or superficial, digital flexor tendon is most likely to occur at about mid-cannon bone. Injury to the deep digital flexor tendon, which is located beneath the superficial tendon, is most likely to occur lower, near the fetlock joint.

5. Now pick up the foot and repeat the examination with the leg flexed. The edges of the tendon will be more difficult to appreciate in this position, as the tendon is now completely relaxed, rather than taut. However, you can practically wrap your fingers around the back of the tendon when the leg is in this position, and you can get a better appreciation for any swelling that might be beginning — the injured portion of the tendon will feel thicker, possibly knotty. The normal tendon is perfectly smooth.

A positive finding in any of the above areas — indistinct tendon edges, filling of the groove in front of the tendon, a "spongy" feeling to the tendon, a change in the appearance of the tendon when viewed from the side (usually a thickening or bulging toward the rear), swelling, heat, or pain — suggests tendon injury. Don't expect to be able to distinguish between an injury of the superficial digital flexor tendon and the deep digital flexor tendon — it's not going to affect your treatment, so it's irrelevant at this point. Realize, too, that if the swelling includes the fetlock joint, there may also be some injury to that joint.

What's going on inside the leg as a result of the injury?

To envision what's going on as a result of the injury, you need to know a little more about what the normal, undamaged tendon looks like. It's basically bundles of bundles — tiny microfibrils are bundled together to form fibrils, fibrils are bundled together to form fascicles, and fascicles are bundled together to form tendon. The bundles are normally kinky, crimped in a uniform zig-zag, like a lazy accordion. During use, the zig-zag crimps straighten out; at rest they spring back to their normal crimp. When the tendon becomes overloaded, the crimps get overstretched and lose their ability to spring back, like an overburdened rubber band. If the overload is severe enough, the tiny inner fibrils begin to slip past each other, and the normally organized structure of the tendon is disrupted.

FIGURE 6.6

Occasionally, bowed tendon occurs in the DDF (deep digital flexor) tendon alone. In this case, the swelling is usually closer to the fetlock joint instead of mid-cannon.

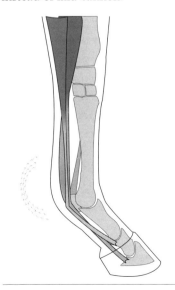

When overload occurs, tiny blood vessels are torn. As they bleed into the structure of the tendon, the blood causes further separation of the tendon's fibrils, furthering the damage and magnifying the pain. Blood also leaks into the space between the tendon and the translucent "sleeve" that encloses it (the tendon sheath). As the body recognizes that the injury has occurred, inflammation develops: tissue fluid oozes into the injured area, causing swelling and heat to develop, further disrupting the fibers of the tendon and distending the tendon sheath. As a rule, the more severe the tissue damage, the faster the inflammation appears. The hemorrhage and tissue fluid escalate the pain and further the damage, and the tendon is even more vulnerable to additional tearing because the separation of fibers weakens it, just as a multifiber rope is weakened when its fibers are separated.

Why is this injury dangerous?

A bowed tendon injury to the superficial digital flexor tendon in the forelimb is the most feared injury among horse trainers. Why? Because of all the common injuries, horses with this type of injury are least likely to return to full performance, and those that do are almost guaranteed to become reinjured.

A healthy tendon is made up of a specific kind of fiber called Type I collagen. When a tendon is injured, the damaged Type I collagen is replaced during the healing process by an inferior fiber called Type III collagen — it's the same kind of collagen found in the tendons of an immature fetus. What's inferior about it? Well, it doesn't have the zig-zag crimps, for one, so it's less elastic than normal Type I collagen. Also, the organization of the fibers is less effective: instead of being set up in systematic, parallel bundles, it's laid down in a haphazard, random fashion — instead of being carefully woven like fine silk, the fibers are mashed together like crafter's felt. To make matters worse, the replacement tendon's fibers are interspersed with "filler" fiber, an amorphous, gloppy mass of fibers thrown into the whole mess to "glue" it together. This "filler" holds the fibrils apart, preventing them from lying in a neat, orderly, parallel fashion alongside each other, and the result is a tendon that is enlarged and lumpy, rather than uniform and smooth.

The good news is, over the ensuing twelve months some remodeling will occur — thanks to the longitudinal pull on the repaired tendon, many of the fibers will re-arrange themselves in a more normal configuration, and some of that messy interfibrillar matrix will be reduced. But they will *never* achieve the same neat organization as in the original, undamaged tendon, and the lumpy interfibrillar matrix will never completely disappear. Besides, the repaired section is still made of inferior Type III fibrils, which will never be crimped like the normal Type I fibrils were. So even under the most ideal of conditions, the repaired tendon is never as strong, never as resilient, never as efficient as before the injury, and it will always be enlarged and misshapen, even if only slightly so. The larger the damaged area, and the more

FIGURE 6.7

In this dramatic case, **the superficial digital flexor tendon, the deep digital flexor tendon, and the suspensory ligament have ruptured completely, allowing the fetlock to drop downward and the toe to cock upward. Complete rupture of any of these structures is most likely to occur from an external blow, such as a kick.**

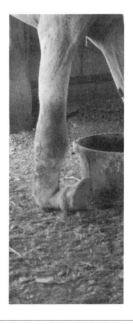

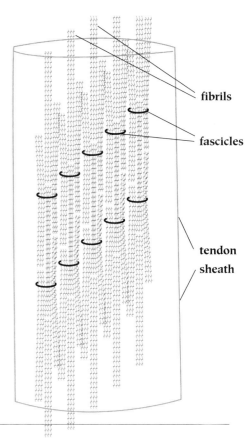

FIGURE 6.8

The normal, healthy tendon is made of bundles of bundles:

bundles of kinky microfibrils form fibrils, bundles of fibrils form fascicles, and bundles of fascicles form tendon.

The tendon, which is very smooth, is encased in a silky sheath, allowing it to glide around joints.

In normal use, the kinks in the micro-fibrils can straighten out when under load, then spring back when the load is lifted, giving the tendon an elastic nature and absorbing the load without disrupting the architecture of the tendon.

Even under the most ideal conditions, the repaired tendon is never as strong, never as resilient, never as good as before the injury. Never.

tissue replacement that is necessary, the more disfigured and dysfunctional the resultant healed area will be. The horse will have an externally noticeable disfigurement and a less flexible, less elastic tendon that is prone to re-injury. Depending on how badly damaged the tendon was to begin with, how quickly and aggressively you treated it, how patient you were in allowing it to heal optimally before asking the horse to work again, and exactly what you ask of your horse, the tendon might eventually be "good enough," but it will never be "as good."

What would the vet do?

Nothing that anyone can do will make the fact of the tendon injury go away. However, the body's response to that injury has the potential of worsening the damage by a full 100% or more — if left to its own devices, the body can more than *double the damage*. A sharp veterinarian will try to halt that extra damage and encourage the existing mess to heal as normally as possible, so that the repaired tendon will mimic the normal tendon as closely as possible in looks, function, and strength. This will require two things:

1. Support the leg to prevent further stretching of the already over-stretched, damaged tendon, and

2. Control hemorrhage and inflammation.

FIGURE 6.9

If stress over-stretches a tendon, the "kinks" will be stretched out of the microfibrils and they'll tear, causing the fibrils to separate and slide apart. If the stress continues, more microfibrils will tear, and more disruption will occur. Bleeding causes further damage, oozing up into the fabric of the fascicles and separating their fibrils even more. Soon the tendon sheath becomes inflamed and swollen.

In this state, the enlarged, swollen, inflamed tendon and sheath are in no condition to withstand the stress of weight-bearing. The stress of continued work frays the fragile fibers, causing more damage, more swelling, more friction...

Clearly, the very first, most important thing to do when a tendon is injured is to relieve it of all duty to prevent further damage.

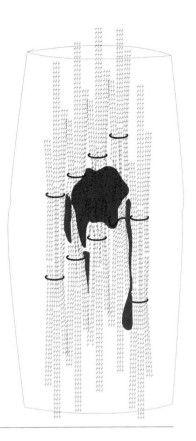

If given the chance — i.e., if called to the scene early enough — the first thing the vet would do is *prevent* inflammation. Not *treat* it, but *prevent* it. To do this, the vet must do the following within fifteen minutes of the injury:

a. A pressure bandage is skillfully applied with a minimum of padding to prevent tissue fluid and blood from entering the damaged area, spreading the tendon fibers apart and filling up the tendon sheath. Skill is required to apply significant pressure without causing more damage by applying that pressure unevenly or in such a way as to inhibit adequate circulation.

b. Diagnostic tools (x-ray, ultrasound) will be used to confirm the diagnosis and make sure there are no additional injuries, such as bone fractures (within the fetlock, or involving the sesamoid bones, for example) or joint damage (most commonly to the fetlock).

c. The leg is iced to slow down the bleeding of tiny torn capillaries in the damaged tendon and further inhibit inflammation. There are several effective methods, including plunging the pressure-wrapped leg into a bucket of ice water, or enveloping the pressure-wrapped leg in any of a number of homemade or commercially available icing apparati (e.g.,the leg of a discarded pair of trousers filled with frozen garden peas, or a chemically activated cold-pack / wrap). The goal is to chill

WARNING!

If a bowed tendon is treated with pain medication only, and no effort is made to immobilize the leg and keep the injured tendon from further stretching injury, the pain relief will encourage the horse to bear full weight on the leg and therefore risk further damage. The pain is a kind of protective measure — it keeps the horse from using the leg fully — and you should not administer any treatment that removes that protection without first supporting the leg to protect the horse against the consequences of that pain relief.

the leg sufficiently to slow the microhemorrhage but to avoid overchilling, which could cause frostbite.

d. To prevent further stretching of the tendon, which will lead to further damage "from the outside," the vet will choose one of several different methods to immobilize the leg. There are three main options: bandage, splint, or cast. Which method is chosen should depend on the severity of the initial injury, and on whether or not the horse will have to be transported to another facility for continued care (e.g., if the vet feels it's necessary to refer the horse to a specialist or to one of the veterinary teaching hospitals affiliated with a veterinary school). If the injury is severe and the horse will have to be transported, splinting or casting should be done to prevent him from abruptly bearing weight on the injured leg while balancing in the trailer. If properly splinted or casted, the leg can still act as a "post" to help balance the horse, but the flexor tendons will be held in a passive, relaxed position to prevent further stretching damage.

e. Antiinflammatory medications are given. Phenylbutazone ("bute") and flunixin meglumine (Banamine®) are popular and very effective. Their effect is to further block inflammation, and to relieve pain (see *WARNING*, previous page).

There's no vet. What should you do?

STEP 1.
Apply a special bandage.

Apply one of the firm pressure bandages specifically designed for bowed tendon injury (see *Chapter 18*). As you're working, remember that you must apply adequate pressure to prevent edema from distending any of the tissues — that's a significant amount of pressure — but you must also be very, very careful not to strangulate or "band" any portion of the leg. You can *cause* a bowed tendon by improperly bandaging a normal leg! Make a smooth, neat bandage with no uneven pressure spots, and don't hesitate to start over if you think it's not going well.

STEP 2.
Chill.

Once the bandage is secure, immediately ice the leg by plunging it, bandage and all, into a bucket of ice water, or by securing bags of crushed ice, frozen peas, or chemical cold packs to the bandaged leg with a track wrap. If you're wrapping cold packs over the outside of the pressure bandage, just leave this chilling method in place until you're ready to apply the support wrap. If you're plunging the leg into ice water, stick closely to this schedule: 5 minutes 'on,' 15 minutes 'off,' 5 minutes 'on,' 15 minutes 'off' and repeat the cycle until you're ready to apply your method of support in the next step.

STEP 3.
Raise the heel.

To alleviate some of the stress on the damaged tendon, apply a wedge to the heel to raise it by 12 to 16 degrees (if you don't happen to have a protractor handy to measure the angles, figure on raising the heel by about an inch, which is the height of a standard rubber door stop). See *Figure 6.10*. Door stops, by the way, make good heel wedges if you don't have the ideal wedge of wood. Use three door stops for an average sized hoof, four if it's a wider hoof. The idea is to raise the heel, not compress the frog. Tape the wedges together into a solid wedge, then tape the whole thing to the heel with duct tape. For more on wedging, see *Chapter 18: The Science and Art of Bandaging.*

If the lameness is extreme and if you'll be moving the horse to a veterinary facility (rather than getting a veterinarian to come to the horse), apply one of the Type IV support methods specifically designed for supporting a bowed tendon in *Chapter 18.* The support method should be applied over the pressure bandage. If the pressure bandage is wet from the icing, replace it with a dry one before applying the support wrap.

STEP 4.
Support the leg.

Now that the leg is safely supported, give phenylbutazone ("bute") paste or gel orally, or Banamine™ injectable intramuscularly. If your horse's lameness is severe, give both. Doses are detailed in *Special Notes 6.7 and 6.8.*

STEP 5.
Give an antiinflammatory.

DMSO? BEWARE!

As we've already discussed, there's some bleeding going on within the damaged tendon. Some authors suggest applying DMSO (dimethylsulfoxide, a clear liquid by-product of the paper industry, used topically as an antiinflammatory) to the freshly injured tendon in order to combat inflammation. In theory this is a great idea, but in practice it can encourage more hemorrhage, because the DMSO causes tiny blood vessels to dilate (expand). If those blood vessels are damaged, as would be the case with a severe injury, dilating them will only allow blood to leak out faster. Your intent is to combat inflammation and thereby *reduce* tissue damage, but what you might actually accomplish is to hasten hemorrhage and thereby *increase* tissue damage. What might have started as a discreet area of injury can become up to three times larger because you've expanded the area of hemorrhage.

Therefore, as a rule, DMSO should not be applied to *fresh* injuries where hemorrhage might still be occurring— its use is cautiously recommended only *after* hemorrhage has been controlled, and the rule of thumb is to allow three days for that to occur.

FIGURE 6.10

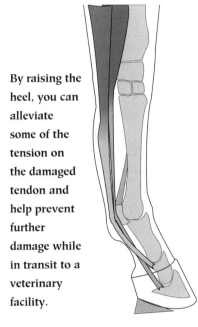

By raising the heel, you can alleviate some of the tension on the damaged tendon and help prevent further damage while in transit to a veterinary facility.

Should you seek veterinary assistance?

Absolutely, and without delay. If the injury is severe, a large number of fibers will have been disrupted, and the tendon sheathing structure will be involved in the resultant inflammation and hemorrhage, upgrading the diagnosis from simple tendinitis to tenosynovitis. Tenosynovitis is more likely to result in the formation of adhesions between that tendon and any nearby structures, including the sheath, other tendons, and other ligaments. Those adhesions are likely to interfere with the normal function

Don't expect the anti-inflammatory medication to make the horse pain-free if he's suffered a serious bowed tendon — he might be very lame for up to six weeks. The medication's role is simply to control the inflammation, which should be under control after two or three days of confinement. After that, time and good nursing care are the prescription, and the "bute" or Banamine™ should be discontinued.

of the tendon, leaving your horse with limited use of the leg after the initial injury has healed. To control the damage that leads to the formation of those adhesions, the vet might opt to put a rigid cast on the leg for three weeks, or surgery might be warranted to drain accumulated blood, clots, and tissue fluid from the tendon sheath. In worst-case tendon damage, such as when the tendon literally tears apart or is severed by an external blow, a surgical option is to insert matrix implants into the remaining tendon tissue to "train" or "guide" the repairing tendon fibrils to grow in a more organized, parallel configuration. Recent work with synthetic implants has even shown promise in getting the replacement tendon to develop with the crimped architecture usually seen only in original, undamaged tendon.

What's the prognosis?

Even completely ruptured tendons can heal, with or without surgery, if given the chance. The prognosis for your horse depends on three things:

1. the severity of the initial damage,

2. how successfully you manage to minimize secondary inflammation and hemorrhage by recognizing the problem early and immediately starting proper preventive measures, and

3. what your plans for the horse were before all this happened.

If you had your sights set on using him as a three-day eventer, and you're unwilling to consider less tendon-strenuous activities for him, his prognosis is guarded, because the stress that activity will place on his second-grade replacement tendons increases the chances that he'll suffer re-injury. But if he's a horse with an active but slightly less strenuous career ahead of him, the prognosis for that kind of future is likely to be better. What will he be capable of doing? Again, it depends on how bad the injury was, and on how successfully you and your veterinarian prevented healing-associated limitations such as adhesions and excess scar tissue. There are successful hunter-jumpers, steeplechasers, barrel racers and endurance racers with bowed tendons, but you can be sure that they're the exceptions, and their injuries were treated immediately and properly as soon as they were recognized.

What about follow-up care?

Until you're able to get him to a veterinarian, keep your horse confined to a small stall where he can lie down if he wants to, and change his bandage frequently, depending on

- how much swelling occurred before you put the bandage on (as the bandage does its anti-swelling magic, the size of the swollen leg decreases and the bandage becomes too loose, requiring that it be re-applied to maintain compression on the

down-sized leg), and

- how skilled you are at bandaging (if you've girdled the leg or applied pressure unevenly, the risk of bandage-induced damage to the leg is significant — if you're unsure of your bandaging ability, you'll need to change the bandage as often as every few hours to make sure you're not doing any damage. Don't take chances. When in doubt, *change the bandage*).

Don't give antiinflammatory medication for longer than one week, and during that week gradually decrease the dose. High doses of antiinflammatory medication given several days in a row absolutely will cause adverse side-effects.

Bucked Shins and Shin Splints

These are conditions of the young adult horse's front cannon bones, due to too much stress on the bones from training or working. The conditions are most often seen in 2- to 5-year olds that work at high speeds and/or with increased concussion to the legs (such as Quarter Horses and Thoroughbreds in race training, young endurance racers, and youngsters in jump training).

What do you see from the outside?

Severe lameness is seen, often appearing the day *after* a heavy workout or race. The front and/or outside surface of one or both forelimb cannon bones is warm and tender to the touch, and in severe cases there will be one or more very sore, pea-sized bumps directly below the knee joint, while the rest of the shin seems to be less ouchy.

FIGURE 6.11

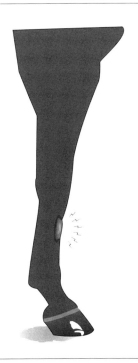

What's going on inside?

In mild cases, the cellophane-like covering over the bone, called the periosteum, is inflamed, which causes heat, swelling, and pain. With increasing severity, the developing bone matrix, frantically trying to add critical thickness to the bone while supporting the horse's training program, becomes involved in the inflammation. In the worst case of bucked shin, the front of the beleaguered cannon bone just below the knee joint develops a network of surface crack-like fractures: this is called *shin splints*. When your horse has shin splints, you'll feel one or more pea-sized bumps on the front of the shin, and the horse will deeply resent having them touched.

Why is this dangerous?

For the most part, the horse will be so sore that he won't allow you to further damage his bones — he'll force you to remove him from the training program and tend to his injuries, and the rest will allow the inflammation and fractures to heal on their own.

Trouble is, trainers or owners who don't know what they're dealing with, or who are in a hurry to get the horse finished and on the circuit, might simply give pain-killing, antiinflammatory medication to relieve the lameness and continue pushing the horse. This can lead to further weakening of the bone and is, in many cases, the underlying reason for racehorses breaking down with dramatic leg fractures on the track — their bones are weak and brittle, and they literally snap under the stress.

What's the most common cause?

Shin splints that were treated with painkillers and put back to work are the underlying cause of many catastrophic leg fractures on the racetrack.

The thickness of the shin bones (the cannon bones) in the horse depends on how hard the bones are used while the horse is maturing — the harder they're worked, the thicker they develop in order to support the load. Once the thickening process is completed, the result is a very strong, tough bone that can stand up to the demands of heavy load-bearing stress and high-speed athletic activity. Until the thickening process is completed, however, the bone is not only less thick than it needs to be, it's even more vulnerable to injury because in the process of becoming thicker, it must first become thinner.

Making the bone thicker is part of what's called the bone remodeling process. In order for the bone to remodel, part of the preexisting bone must be removed to make way for new, thicker layers. Bone-eating cells called osteoclasts move in and literally eat away part of the preexisting bone, then bone-building cells called osteoblasts move in and begin building a matrix to accept thicker layers of new bone. Unfortunately, this incomplete bone-factory-in-progress is extremely weak and vulnerable to damage from training stress. It's ironic: the stress is needed in order to stimulate the bone to thicken, and yet that very stress can damage the bone during the remodeling process. Work the horse too hard during this period, and you'll cause damage ranging from mild inflammation to actual microfractures. Work him too little, and his bones won't thicken enough. It's the ultimate trainer's challenge.

What would the vet do?

The diagnosis of bucked shins is usually obvious, but radiographs should be taken in order to grade the severity of the condition and to make sure there aren't any other problems going on at the same time:

Level I Bucked Shins The leg is warm and sore to palpation, but there are no radiographic changes seen (i.e., the x-rays look normal).

Level II Bucked Shins The leg is warm and sore to palpation, and radiographs reveal mild inflammation of the periosteum (the edges of the bone look somewhat blurry)

The leg is warm and sore to palpation, and radiographs reveal advanced inflammation of the periosteum (a broad section of the bone's edge looks thick and "fuzzy").

Level III Bucked Shins

The leg is warm and sore to palpation, has distinct pea-sized bumps that are easily found just under the knee joint, and radiographs reveal stress or shear type fractures in the surface of the bone cortex.

Level IV Bucked Shins ("Shin Splints")

Veterinary treatment of bucked shins includes immediate icing, firm support bandaging, daily hydrotherapy, antiinflammatory medication (usually phenylbutazone) for three to five days, stall rest (for up to two weeks, depending on the severity of the case), and some major changes to the training program. Some veterinarians advocate surgical treatment for shin splints — under anesthesia the "angry" area of bone is scrubbed and flushed to remove debris and tiny chips of bone. The added expense of the surgery is usually offset by a shorter convalescent time.

Newer treatments that might be included: "cold laser" therapy, ultrasound therapy, and magnetic therapy. These therapies require expensive equipment and it's still too soon to say how effective they are, but they do show great promise in selected cases. Their aim is to speed the recovery process and get the horse back to training with a minimum of convalescent time.

The thickness of the shin (cannon) bones in the horse depends on how hard those bones are worked while the horse is maturing — the more stress they're exposed to during that formative period, the thicker they develop in order to support the load.

There's no vet. What should you do?

The diagnosis is generally pretty obvious, and aside from taking radiographs, which are done mainly to confirm the diagnosis and assess the severity of the case, most of the non-surgical treatments the veterinarian would do for bucked shins are things you can do yourself.

Emergency treatment:

Ice the affected legs by plunging in a bucket of ice water for five minutes, or applying packs of crushed ice or hosing with very cold water for five minutes at a time every 20 minutes.

STEP 1. Ice.

Meanwhile, give oral phenylbutazone (see *Special Note 6.7* for dose) daily for up to three days or until the horse is no longer lame at a walk and shows minimal or no tenderness on palpation of the shin, whichever happens first.

STEP 2. "Bute."

Dry the legs and apply a Class II bandage from coronary band to knee joint (see *Chapter 18*).

STEP 3. Wrap.

Stall rest.

STEP 4. Confine.

Follow-up care:

STEP 5.
Water therapy.

Daily for the next two days, undress the leg, treat it with an invigorating stream of cold water or a cold water whirlpool bath for ten minutes, then dry and re-apply the bandage.

STEP 6.
DMSO.

Beginning after Day 3 (but not before): after the water therapy, paint the leg with an equal mixture of nitrofurazone ointment and DMSO liquid or gel, and wrap the painted leg with a soft Type II bandage (*do not apply* Cool-Cast™ *after treating with DMSO — see Special Note 6.9*). Re-bandage daily until swelling is completely and consistently gone.

STEP 7.
Adjust the training program.

Return to work gradually and check both shins often for heat and tenderness. Adjust the training program to push the horse adequately for conditioning without risking excessive shin stress. Remember — you have to push him in order for his bones to thicken and strengthen, but there's a fine line between pushing enough and pushing too much.

Should you seek veterinary assistance?

It's generally not critical, as long as you're sure there isn't something else going on besides the bucked shins. As a rule, classic cases of bucked shins respond quickly and in an uncomplicated way to the above treatment protocol, and if your horse's response is incomplete or in some way complicated, you should seek veterinary confirmation of your diagnosis and additional treatment options. Veterinary follow-up is also helpful in judging recovery and determining when, and to what extent, to return to training.

SPECIAL NOTE 6.9

DMSO is instantly absorbed into the bloodstream through the skin — that's why you notice an "oyster" or "garlic" taste in your mouth if you touch the liquid without gloves. Therefore, you must not use any liniments, blisters, or medicated dressings such as Cool-Cast™ along with DMSO — their active ingredients can be dangerous if carried into the bloodstream by the DMSO.

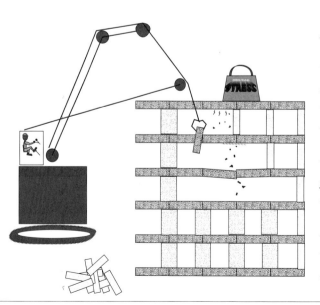

Training the youngster is a delicate balancing act. Just as in remodeling a house, the old walls must be torn down before new ones can be erected in their place. Before young bones-in-training complete their remodeling process in preparation for a life of athletic competition, they go through a period when they are thinner, weaker than they were before training began.

"Popped Knees" (injuries to the carpus)

FIGURE 6.12

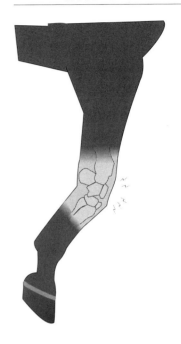

This is a complex collection of different injuries to bone and/or soft tissue structures within the knee joint of one or both forelimbs. Even though a bony fracture is much different from a soft tissue injury in terms of ultimate treatment, distinguishing these types of injury is usually impossible without technical support such as x-ray, ultrasound, and possibly even arthroscopic exploratory surgery. Therefore, from the horse owner's point of view, all severe injuries of the knee joint are lumped together and handled as though they were a worst-case scenario until a detailed veterinary examination can prove otherwise. The important thing from the emergency treatment point of view is recognizing that the knee joint is the focus of the horse's problem.

What you see from the outside

The horse will "walk wide," swinging the leg to the outside to move it forward without bending the sore knee. The involved joint might be puffy (called "hygroma") and warm, depending on the severity and freshness of the injury and depending on whether it involves bone or soft tissue or both. In most cases, the problem is obvious when the foot is picked up and the joint is forced to flex — the horse will flinch or otherwise display a painful response. In the normal horse, you should be able to bend the leg to easily touch the heel to the elbow. The horse with a sore knee will tense the leg and prevent this flexion if it hurts, and the lameness will be exaggerated temporarily when you put the foot back down. Other signs: the horse might resent having the joint manipulated, and the joint might be tender to the touch.

What causes knee injuries?

Cartilage erosion and arthritis are usually gradual and chronic and will not be discussed here. There are three main types of sudden, severe knee lameness common in performance horses:

1. bone fractures,
2. ligament strains, and
3. inflammation of the joint capsule.

Fatigue plays a major role in knee injuries, and the activities that predispose to each type of injury are described below. Severe knee injuries are often a combination of injury types.

The most dramatic knee joint injuries involve chip and/or crushing fractures of one or more bones inside the carpal joint. With fatigue, the muscles allow the carpal bones to move out of proper alignment when the joint is stressed, and since they're supposed to interlock perfectly during maximal load, fractures are highly likely when

CARPAL CHIP FRACTURES

The joint is usually hot, swollen, sensitive to the touch, and sensitive to being held in the flexed position. Lameness is usually obvious at a walk.

they're out of position and 1,100 pounds of mass are barreling down the leg at high speed. The most common victims are youngsters in training, especially heavy-bodied, inherently fast-sprinting Quarter Horses that can pour on the speed early in their careers, without prior conditioning. Youngsters in jump training are at risk, particularly when asked to jump before they've developed adequate strength in their legs. Carpal chip fractures are frequent findings in horses that run downhill, an activity that is common during endurance races, delivering a concussive beating to the knees. Weekend warriors' horses are at risk because of lack of conditioning and marshmallow-soft muscles that are unable to absorb much of the stress of load-bearing.

INFLAMED CARPAL LIGAMENTS

The joint may or may not be swollen and hot, it's usually not sensitive to the touch, but it is sensitive to being held in the flexed position.

One of the most common soft tissue injuries in the knee joint is inflammation of the ligaments that hold the rows of carpal bones in position. This is most often seen in youngsters in early training and is a result of stress on the knee joints from a training program that's too strenuous too soon. Rather than concussive insults, it's quick changes in direction, jack-rabbit starts, sliding stops, and extended trots that are most often implicated — any moves that tend to twist, torque, or bend the little cube-shaped bones out of their neat, orderly rows, or that ask the hinge-like joint to overextend (common in youthful, poorly executed extended trots) or bend sideways (common in young cutting horses).

INFLAMED JOINT CAPSULE

The joint is hot and swollen, sore to the touch, and the lameness worsens after the leg is held in flexion.

The other common non-bony carpal joint injury is inflammation of the joint capsule, also known as synovitis/capsulitis. It is the result of excessive stress on the joint under load, particularly when the ligaments are loose (I hate to sound like a broken record, but it's common in youngsters pushed beyond their early abilities). From the outside, the symptoms are the same as you'd see with a chip fracture, and to make matters even more confusing, in some (but not all) cases synovitis is a symptom of a chip fracture. Only diagnostic imaging can tell you the bottom line.

What would the vet do?

SPECIAL NOTE 6.10

Injecting a joint with a steroid medication used to be a popular, almost routine, treatment for "popped knees." It should never, ever be done to your horse unless diagnostic work has been done to ensure there's no fracture and no infection, in which steroids would be like fuel to a fire.

The carpal joint is a complicated Pandora's box, and getting a clear x-ray of what's happening inside the joint is no easy task — the bones are many and small, fractures can be tiny chips hiding in remote, difficult to see corners, and injuries of the ligaments can create symptoms so severe that you'd swear there's a fracture in there somewhere — but there isn't. In some cases, the final diagnosis can only be achieved by exploratory arthroscopic surgery.

The treatment and prognosis hang heavily on the veterinarian's ability to get an accurate diagnosis. Therefore, the bulk of his/her efforts, as well as the bulk of your expense, will be spent on getting that diagnosis. Fractures may or may not require surgery, depending on their extent and on their location within the joint, and surgery might involve removing the chip, or various methods employed to put it back into place (bone screw, wire, pin, cast). Whether or not surgery is done, stall rest and medications to minimize swelling and inflammation are an essential part of the recovery process.

There's no vet. What should you do?

Strict stall confinement for 48 hours is a must to further limit damaging forces to the injured leg. As soon as it's safe to do so (the leg is well protected and the quickest route has been mapped out), the horse should be transported to a competent equine orthopedist for a specific diagnosis.

STEP 1.
Confine.

Ice the knee, using crushed ice packs, bags of frozen peas, chemical cold packs, or cold water rinses. Ice on: 5 minutes. Ice off: 15 minutes. Repeat the cycle for 48 hours.

STEP 2.
Ice.

Apply a Class III or Class IV knee bandage to limit movement and minimize swelling (see *Chapter 18*). Until the exact nature of the injury is known, it's critical that further damage to the inside of the joint be prevented by immobilizing the leg. Shredded ligaments, torn cartilages, and sharp bone fragments can combine to make the problem much worse if the horse is permitted to move the leg freely.

STEP 3.
Immobilize.

An intramuscular injection of Banamine™ can keep inflammation and its by-products from worsening the damage, and its pain-killing action will help to make the horse more comfortable. See *Special Note 6.8* for dose recommendations. Do not give this medication if for some reason you can't properly bandage the leg — if you relieve the pain without restricting leg movement, you set the stage for massive additional damage.

STEP 4.
Give an
antiinflammatory.

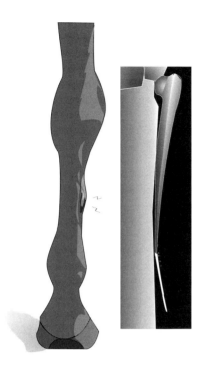

Splint bone injury

When you look at a horse's skeleton, it might appear that the thin, rudimentary splint bones that run down either side of the shin have no function. But because of their close association with tendons and ligaments, and because they're located in an area of the leg where they're virtually unprotected against external trauma, they're prone to injury and can cause significant lameness. The injury can be as mild as simple irritation, or as severe as fracture, and the severity of the resultant lameness will depend on the type and location of the injury. What you typically think of as "splints" in young, growing horses might cause some tenderness to the touch and swelling of the space between the splint bone and the cannon bone, but they're generally considered part of the normal maturation process and are rarely associated with lameness, and therefore they will not be considered here. Rather, traumatic injury to the splint bone in the adult horse will be the focus of this discussion.

What you see from the outside

Depending on the severity of the injury, there will be swelling and pain starting along the side and toward the front of the shin, where the splint bone joins with the cannon bone. With increasing severity and fracture, the area of swelling and pain can extend toward the back of the cannon bone and involve the entire body of the splint bone.

What's the cause of splint bone injuries?

Splint bone fractures occur most commonly in the forelimbs of older performance horses that already have some inflammation of the suspensory ligament. Fractures at the low (distal) end of the splint bone most often occur when the leg is under heavy load, the fetlock is extended down to the ground, and the ligaments connecting to the sesamoid bones at the back of the fetlock joint are pulling hard on the splint bone. Fractures at the high (proximal) end of the splint bone, up nearer the knee joint, most often occur from external trauma such as a kick, and in half of these cases, there's an associated open wound through the skin.

What would the vet do?

Fractures of the far (distal) end of the splint bones usually heal on their own with two to three months of stall rest and a slow controlled return to work. The recovery period is significantly shortened if the broken-off piece of splint bone is surgically removed. Higher fractures leave a bigger broken-off piece that must either be reattached surgically or removed in order to expect uncomplicated healing. The typical veterinary approach to this type of injury would be to secure a definitive diagnosis, perform the surgery, then prescribe stall rest and regular bandage changes followed by a gradual return to work.

There's no vet. What should you do?

The diagnosis should be easy to make, particularly if there's an open wound from external trauma over the splint bone, and it should be obvious that the splint bone area is where the horse is most resentful of palpation. Gentle probing with your fingertips may reveal crepitus, a bubbly, popping sensation that usually indicates fracture.

Ice the affected leg by plunging it in ice water for five minutes at a time, or by applying packs of crushed ice, frozen peas, or chemical cool packs, 5 minutes "on", 15 minutes "off", for up to two hours.

STEP 1.
Ice.

If the skin is broken over the splint bone injury (e.g., if the injury occured as a result of a kick), clean and dress the wound as you would any superficial laceration (see *Chapter 7*).

STEP 2.
Attend to any open wounds.

Dry the leg and apply Cool-Cast™ from the coronary band to the knee joint. If there is an open wound, be sure to cover it first with its own bandage— do not apply Cool-Cast™ directly over an open wound.

STEP 3.
Wrap.

Give oral phenylbutazone (see *Special Note 6.7* for dose) daily for up to three days or until the horse is no longer lame at a walk and shows minimal or no tenderness on palpation of the splint, whichever happens first.

STEP 4.
Give an antiinflammatory.

Check tetanus vaccination status and update it: give tetanus toxoid if the last toxoid was given within the past six months. If the last toxoid was given more than six months ago, give tetanus toxoid in one location and tetanus antitoxin in another. See *Special Note 6.5* for information on the potential hazards of giving tetanus antitoxin.

STEP 5.
TETANUS

Confine the horse to a stall to prevent further injury until the splint is resolved either conservatively or by surgery. Even if your horse's splint bone injury is one that might require surgery, that decision can be made at any time — there's no rush.

STEP 6.
Confine.

Should you seek veterinary assistance?

If rapid recovery is important for the fastest return to work, x-rays and veterinary examination should be done as soon as possible to determine whether this particular injury will heal faster with surgical treatment. If you opt to go it alone, be advised that if the horse is not significantly better after the above treatment and one week of confinement, you've got something worse going on. Don't take chances — get the horse checked out.

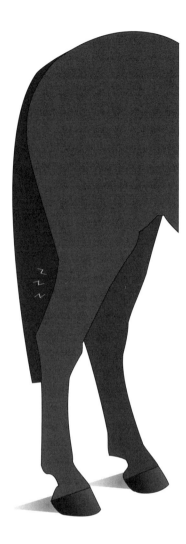

THE UPPER LEG

Tibial stress fracture

This is a common but little-known condition of the hindlimbs in young horses in training. In fact, this condition could be the most misdiagnosed lameness in the training Thoroughbred horse, as it tends to be overlooked and tossed into the no-man's-land of confusing lamenesses called "sore stifles." In essence, it's the hindlimb's version of bucked shins, only instead of occurring on the front-outside surface of the cannon bone, it occurs on the back-inside surface of the tibia (the bone just above the hock).

What you see

Victims show a sudden onset of stiff, stilted, shortened gait in one or both hind limbs. Because they move their legs stiffly, it appears that they wish to protect their stifles, as though it hurts to flex them. Therefore, horses with tibial stress fracture are often misdiagnosed as having "sore stifles."

What's going on inside

The problem is in the tibia, the bone that lies between the hock and the stifle. The bone of the tibia in the young animal in training undergoes many of the same changes in response to stress as does the cannon bone in the front leg — it thickens and strengthens as the animal matures through his training regimen. Paradoxically, the process of thickening the bone requires that the bone first be weakened by bone-eating cells called osteoclasts, which move in and remove layers of bone in preparation for the laying-down of extra layers of new, thicker bone. Bone-building cells called osteoblasts then move in, erecting a matrix upon which extra layers of new, thicker bone will be laid down. Unfortunately, until this thickening process is completed, the bone is weaker and more vulnerable to stress-related injury. Excessive training stress during this period of time can damage the weakened bone, causing injury with a range of severity from mild inflammation of the cellophane-like periosteal coating over the bone, to actual microfractures on the bone's surface.

What would the vet do?

Radiographs are taken to confirm the diagnosis, and to dispel all the well-meaning but misdirected advice of fellow horsemen who swear that the problem is in the stifles.

Once the diagnosis of tibial stress fracture is confirmed, treatment is simple: stall rest. For how long? It depends on the severity of the damage, but it'll range from one to four months. Clearly, this injury takes longer to heal than shin splints that can generally return to training in 2 weeks.

There's no vet. What should you do?

You can confirm the diagnosis on your own by two simple tests.

STEP 1.
Confirm your diagnosis.

a. Pick up the hind limb and slide your thumb under the muscle bellies that run down the back of the tibia (the bone just above the hock). The horse with tibial stress fracture exhibits pain when you press on the bone here.

b. Knock on the inside surface of the bone with your knuckles: he'll resent this too.

Withdraw from competition/training and rest the horse. Unfortunately, for adequate healing in severe cases, the rest period is extended: 90 to 120 days. You can assess your horse for healing by repeating the tests in step 1 every week while the horse is confined, then repeating the tests daily while gradually returning him to training.

STEP 2.
Rest the horse.

Should you seek veterinary assistance?

Yes, because without technical diagnostic support, you can't be sure that the stifle joint hasn't been injured. If tibial stress fracture is confirmed, that same technical support can be helpful in assessing the horse's recovery and response to resumed training.

Superficial Lacerations & Barbed Wire Cuts

A superficial laceration is a tear or cut in the skin and superficial subcutaneous tissues.

Lacerations can be neat slices, as they often are when resulting from sharp edges of sheet metal; or jagged, as is often the case when a sleek, smooth leg tangles with barbed wire. Skin caught on a protruding nail often suffers the most destructive type of laceration : the tear.

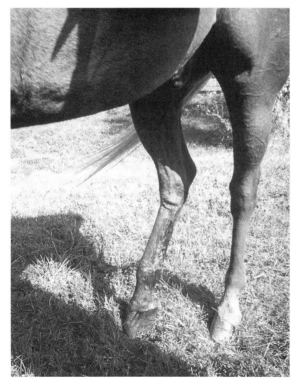

What you see from the outside

Fresh lacerations can look very dramatic, even when they're minor. Regardless of the severity of tissue damage, the predominant thing the eye registers at first is BLOOD — trickling, streaming, gushing or spurting, depending on what structures have been injured, the extent of the damage, and the general condition of the horse at the time of the injury. If the horse had been exercising at the time, or if he is agitated or nervous now (as you'd expect him to be after being caught up in barbed wire), his blood pressure will be elevated and the blood will flow faster (see *Special Note 7.3*).

Often it isn't until the bleeding is controlled that the extent of structural damage can be judged. Initial lameness from a laceration will depend less on the depth of the cut and more on how long it's been since it happened, because the pain is more a function of the i ﬂammation that comes *after* the laceration, rather than the laceration itself. How fast that inflammation develops depends on the severity and extent of the injury, where on the body it occurred, and how dirty or contaminated it is — the deeper, wider and dirtier the wound, and the closer it is to moveable weight-bearing structures within the leg, the faster the inflammation (and associated pain) will show up.

Why is this sort of injury dangerous?

Don't be fooled into thinking "superficial" means "not serious." Blood loss can be significant in superficial leg lacerations. The major digital artery and vein in the pastern and cannon bone area, and the large superficial blood vessels higher in the leg can readily permit a dangerous volume of blood to be lost when the type of injury, the agitation of the horse, and the high blood pressure and increased blood volume of strenuous exercise all conspire to push the blood out faster than it can clot.

How much blood loss is dangerous? Actually, it depends less on how *much* blood is lost, and more on how *fast* it is lost. A horse can lose gallons of blood by a slow trickle and still be safe, while less bleeding can be fatal if it occurs more quickly (see *Special Note 7.1*).

What would the vet do?

The sharp veterinarian will concentrate first on getting the hemorrhage under control by applying a pressure bandage directly over the wound and encouraging horse and humans to calm down. This will allow the horse's blood pressure to drop so the damaged blood vessels can contract and the leaking blood can clot and plug up the holes. The horse in general, rather than just the injured leg, will then be examined to determine whether he's in danger of shock from blood loss. If his cardiovascular system is determined to be well adjusted to the situation after he calms down, he'll be either sedated or anesthetized so that the wound can be properly inspected and treated. Only then will the vet attend to the wound itself, by doing the following:

- Ice the injured area to further slow hemorrhage, to retard or halt the inflammatory process, and to slow down the metabolism of adjacent, undamaged tissues so they'll need less blood to stay alive. If the hemorrhage is severe, the vet might decide to surgically tie off the severed blood vessels.

- Give a non-steroidal antiinflammatory medication such as Banamine™ and/or "bute" to further slow the inflammatory process.

- Shave away the hair and irrigate the injured area to flush out embedded debris and shreds of dead tissue.

- If any portion of the wound seems very deep or is suspected of involving vital structures, the vet might probe that section with a sterile metal instrument and take an x-ray to judge the extent of the wound.

- Scrub and close the wound by suturing, gluing, stapling, and/or bandaging.

SPECIAL NOTE 7.1

HOW MUCH BLOOD LOSS IS TOO MUCH?

The *rate* at which the blood is lost is as important, if not more so, than the *volume* that is lost. If the blood leaks out slowly over a three-day period, a horse can survive losing almost 2/3 of all his blood. Over only 24 hours, the loss of 1/3 of all his blood can be fatal. If the bleeding is faster than that, the loss of as little as 1/10 the total blood volume can be life threatening.

How much blood does your horse have? See *Special Note 7.2*.

SPECIAL NOTE 7.2

HOW MUCH BLOOD DOES YOUR HORSE HAVE?

Depending on his state of health and athletic condition, about 7 to 8% of your horse's body weight consists of circulating blood. Since your horse is a performance animal, his blood volume is probably 8% (athletes have more blood than inactive individuals). Check this chart for an estimate of your horse's total blood volume.

Body Weight	Blood Volume
800 lb	8 gallons
900 lb	8.5 gallons
1000 lb	9 gallons
1100 lb	10 gallons
1200 lb	11 gallons
1300 lb	12 gallons
1400 lb	13 gallons

SPECIAL NOTE 7.3

Hemorrhage is riskier when a laceration occurs during exercise because the body does 3 things to help cope with the demands of work:

1. The heart pumps faster and harder, moving more blood with each stroke.
2. The blood vessels in "non-essential" areas constrict so the hard-working legs, heart and lungs can have more blood.
3. The spleen, which is like a huge sponge holding "extra" blood for high-demand situations, squeezes its supply into the circulation, adding as much as 3 more gallons of blood to the system.

These steps help the fit horse keep up his pace without getting fatigued, but they can also turn an otherwise manageable laceration into a dangerous "gusher."

- Apply a pressure bandage or combination pressure/support splint.
- Check on the horse's tetanus immunization status and give tetanus toxoid and/or tetanus antitoxin as appropriate.
- Decide whether continued antiinflammatory and/or antibiotic therapy is warranted, based on how severe the injury is, how dirty it was, and whether complications will be expected.

There's no vet. What should you do?

If the hemorrhage from your horse's injury is a major concern, focus your initial efforts on steps 1-4 below, and do not continue to step 5 until you're satisfied that the issue of major bleeding is put to rest.

If hemorrhage is not a significant concern with this particular injury, you can progress through the first four steps quickly, ignore the prescribed waiting period, and continue directly to step 5.

STEP 1.

Pressure to the wound, calm to the horse

If it appears that there has been a lot of blood lost already and it's showing no signs of slowing down, focus on getting the bleeding stopped.

a. Quickly but carefully apply a Hemorrhage-Class bandage with pressure evenly and directly exerted over the wound(s) (see *Chapter 18*). Be sure to extend the bandage well above and below the wounded area.

b. Calm the horse to get his blood pressure back down to earth and to get his "emergency reserve" blood to return to the spleen, thereby lowering his total blood volume by up to three gallons (see *Special Note 7.3*) — as long as he's anxious, that extra splenic blood will remain in circulation, potentially adding to the puddle soaking into your bandage and accumulating on the ground. Remain calm yourself so as not to transmit your anxiety to the horse. Do not attempt to calm him with a sedative or tranquilizer — these drugs can cause a *sudden* drop in blood pressure which, when combined with significant blood loss, can make him faint. Instead, try a gentle massage or acupressure (see pages 124–125).

    c. Ice the bandaged leg, by one of the following two methods:

- incorporate a pack of crushed ice, a bag of frozen corn or peas, or a chemical cool-pak in the bandage, or

- toss a gallon of crushed ice into a five-gallon bucket, fill it up with water, and plunge the bandaged leg into the chilly mix for five minutes at a time, every 20 minutes, for one to two hours.

SPECIAL NOTE 7.5

If you're applying icepacks to bare skin, or if you're plunging the bandaged leg into ice water, do not exceed the ice-on time or you could cause frostbite.

    5 minutes "on," 15 minutes "off": that's the drill.

Confine the horse to a small area where it's quiet, dark and cool, and leave the pressure bandage on for one full hour. If it becomes soaked through with blood during that hour, *do not* take it off to apply a dry bandage — this will only give the hemorrhage new life. Simply apply another layer of pressure bandage on top of the existing, soaked bandage, pulling it snugly while distributing the pressure evenly, being careful not to create any tourniquet or constriction effects.

    Do not attempt to hose the blood from the leg or wipe it from the bandage — leave it undisturbed so that the horse will remain unaroused and the damaged blood vessels will have a chance to build a sturdy clot without risk of that clot being dislodged by a sudden rise in blood pressure or by premature manipulation.

    If you fear that the blood already lost has already put your horse in danger of shock from low blood pressure, do not delay — as soon as you've got the pressure bandage secured and the horse confined, go find someone who can try to locate a veterinarian and bring him/her to your horse's side, if at all possible.

SPECIAL NOTE 7.6

WHY ICE AN INJURY?

The damaged area can more than double in size when adjacent tissues, not involved in the initial trauma, die because of impaired blood supply (from blood vessels that are torn or collapsed under the pressure of the swelling). Chilling the tissues slows their metabolism, which temporarily decreases their need for blood and oxygen. This can keep them alive until you can get the crisis under control.

SPECIAL NOTE 7.4

Do not give any tranquilizers or sedatives — not only will they lower his blood pressure too quickly and increase the risk that he might faint, they also can make the horse unsteady on his feet and lead to sudden, illogical, and/or aggressive reactions to your ministrations that could get you hurt and get his bleeding started all over again.

STEP 2.

Confine

SPECIAL NOTE 7.7

WHAT'S THE RUSH?

For the first 3 hours after an injury, the dirt, debris, and bacteria on the wound remain on the surface where they can be removed physically when the wound is cleaned. Between 3 - 6 hours, the bacteria begin to migrate deeper in search of a suitable place to set up an infection. Once they've penetrated, no amount of scrubbing can remove them without removing the tissue they've already invaded.

STEP 3.
Wait 1 hour, then re-assess

If you are unable to get help, re-assess the horse's general condition after the bandage has been on for one full hour. (For more detail on how to perform and interpret these tests, see *Chapter 19: Vital Signs*.)

- Are his gums dramatically pale? (Compare to another horse if you're unsure)

- Does he seem weak, wobbly, or "spacey?"

- Place your hand under his chin and push upward so that his eyes will roll down, exposing the whites — do they look absolutely opaque and ghostly white, possibly even blue-tinged, devoid of any of the thin blood vessels usually visible at the margin of the colored part of the eye?

- Check his capillary refill time by blanching a spot on his gums with finger pressure, then counting how many seconds ("one thousand one, one thousand two") it takes for that spot to re-pink — is it longer than three seconds?

- pinch a little "tent" of skin on the side of his neck where it joins with the shoulder. Does the tent remain standing for more than 1/2 second?

Generally, the more significant the blood loss, the fewer "bloodshot" vessels are visible in the whites of the eyes.

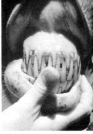

    If your answer to these questions is "yes," your horse may have lost sufficient blood to be in a fragile general state, at risk of fainting or going into shock from low blood pressure. In this case, do not attempt to tend to his wounds, since removing the bandage might restart the hemorrhage. Again, if at all possible, get professional help to come to you — the horse might need emergency surgery (to tie off the damaged blood vessels), and/or he might need a blood transfusion. It's better not to try to move him if you think he may be on the verge of shock.

STEP 4.
Focus on the whole horse

If it's absolutely impossible to find help, concentrate on keeping the horse calm, keeping the wound undisturbed, and getting some water and nourishment into your horse. In other words, focus on the horse, let the pressure bandage and ice work on the wound.

- Offer two buckets of water, side by side: one plain, and one containing powdered electrolytes designed for endurance horses. Place the buckets directly in front of him so he can reach them without moving.

- Offer good quality grass hay (avoid rich grains right now — he's too upset, and you don't want him to colic on top of everything else).

- Offer loose salt to lick.

Assessment of gum color and capillary refill time can indicate the seriousness of blood loss.

(For more on how to do this, see *Chapter 19: Vital Signs*).

    If you have any doubt about his general condition, wait another hour and repeat the examination detailed in Step #3 before moving on.

If, on the other hand, the horse's general condition seems fine, and/or you estimate that he lost no more than a quart of blood by the time you successfully got the bleeding stopped (which, for a horse, is a trivial loss), chances are that his general condition is solid, and you can begin to attend to the wound.

Be absolutely sure the bleeding is stopped and the horse's general condition is stable (take your time — you've got up to three hours if you need them; see *Special Note 7.7*). When you're satisfied, remove the bandage slowly and carefully so as not to stir up the tissues and get the bleeding started again. If the blood in the bandage has dried and glued the fabric together, soak it first with cool water to melt the "glue" and keep the bandage from sticking to the wound. Otherwise, pulling it off might disturb the clot and start the bleeding again (although it's unlikely to be the magnitude of bleeding that you saw in the beginning). Unravel the bandage, rather than cut it off — it's gentler, and it'll relieve the pressure on the leg gradually, rather than suddenly. In this way, you'll be much less likely to dislodge the main blood clots that have sealed off the damaged blood vessels. A little oozing and trickling of blood is expected — what you're trying to avoid is the firehose gush.

Gently irrigate the wound. Depending on the size of the injury and on what equipment you have available, you can either use a garden hose and clean, cool water, or you can use a trigger-type spray bottle containing a homemade saline solution (see *Special Note 7.8* for recipe). If you use the hose, be sure to do a "final rinse" with the salt solution.

To irrigate a large or badly contaminated wound, run a soft, non-aggressive stream of clean, cool water over the entire leg, starting *below* the wound and gradually working your way *up*, across the wound, then *above* it. The horse will resent the touch of the water at first and try to evade it, but be persistent and continue your water massage even when the leg is held up — eventually your horse will decide that the water stream feels soothing, just as your foot eventually finds a too-hot bath to finally be acceptable. This is the result of a nerve fiber reaction called *tempe* — at first, the raw nerves scream with pain, but after repeatedly firing and firing, stimulated by the touch of the water stream, they become numb, immune to the stimulus, and they stop firing. It's a form of natural anesthesia. You'll know when this has happened with your horse — he'll set his foot back down on the ground, lower his formerly raised, alerted head, and let out a relaxed sigh. Now you can get some real work done.

Begin increasing the intensity of the water stream so that it will loosen and dislodge any shreds or tags of gelatinous serum, debris, congealed blood, and dead tissue from the wound.

There's a good reason for doing this: bacteria in a contaminated wound adhere to the tissues by electrostatic charge. In order to get those bacteria off the wound, you must lavage the wound with enough pressure to dislodge them. It doesn't take much — just enough to gently but assertively strike the tissues, about

STEP 5.

Got the bleeding stopped? Okay. Remove the bandage.

SPECIAL NOTE 7.8

Homemade saline solution for wound irrigation:

Mix 1 tsp table salt in 1 quart cool, clean water

STEP 6.

Irrigate

The trigger-type sprayer provides sufficient water pressure to dislodge superficial bacteria that cling to a wound and threaten to cause infection.

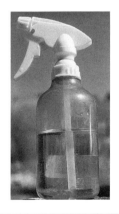

For stubborn grit or ground-in debris, a gentle cleansing with an infant's toothbrush and a surgical soap is helpful.

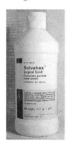 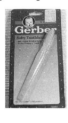

seven psi (pounds per square inch) of pressure.

Continue lavaging until the entire wound is absolutely clean — any cleaning that you do later will be much less effective (see *Special Note 7.7*). If necessary, clean the nooks and crannies of the wound with a very soft infant's toothbrush dipped in Betadine™ Scrub (the kind that lathers) or Solvahex™, and rinse thoroughly afterwards.

Douse the wound with a final rinse of the saline solution. This will help to draw swelling out of the tissues, and it will remove any traces of soap and serum from the area. If you don't have a trigger-type spray bottle, you can use a 60-cc syringe with a blunted 18-gauge needle.

STEP 7.
Dry

Press the leg dry with clean, absorbent towels — don't rub. If it's a sunny day, allow it to air-dry for ten minutes or so. Dab and press any freshly oozed blood with clean stacks of 4 x 4 gauze sponges, being sure to use a fresh, clean stack for each dab.

STEP 8.
Give an antiinflammatory for severe injuries.

If this was a particularly nasty or extensive wound, then while the leg is air-drying, and if your vet entrusted you with a prescription for oral phenylbutazone ("bute"), give a dose now (for dose recommendations, see *Special Note 7.10*). If you have no bute, but you do have Banamine™, you can give the Banamine™ instead. Again, this is only indicated if the wound was severe or very contaminated. See *Special Note 7.11* for dose recommendations.

STEP 9.
Tetanus

Check the horse's tetanus vaccination status and administer a toxoid booster or an antitoxin injection as appropriate (see *Chapter 6 Special Note 6.5* for information on the potential hazards of giving tetanus antitoxin). Avoid the use of "preventive" antibiotics — the best way to prevent infection is to get the wound absolutely clean and keep it that way (see *Chapter17*).

STEP 10.
Press disturbed tissues into their rightful places.

If there are any flaps or tags of tissue hanging out of position, press them firmly where they belong — don't snip them off. It's very difficult, at this early stage, to know which sections of damaged tissue will die because of the extent of their damage, and which will re-attach themselves to their former beds and live to see another day. Tissue that dies can always be removed later, and small sections of dead tissue often fall off on their own. If you're having trouble getting flaps of skin to stay where you press them, "glue" them into position with a gob of antibacterial ointment.

STEP 11.
Dress the wound.

Cover the entire wound with a single layer of gauze sponges that you've impregnated with the antibacterial ointment. Do not use a wound powder or aerosol spray. Use as many pads as necessary to cover the entire wound, and rely on the lightweight nature of the single-layer gauze, as well as the tackiness of the ointment, to "glue" this layer into place.

ASKING FOR TROUBLE:

Beware of lacerations in these locations! Don't be fooled into believing that significant blood loss won't happen if the cut is superficial. The targets mark areas where large blood vessels are located just under the skin, with no "meat" covering them for protection against injury. In the exercising horse, lacerations in these areas can actually lead to potentially fatal hemorrhage unless quick, appropriate action is taken.

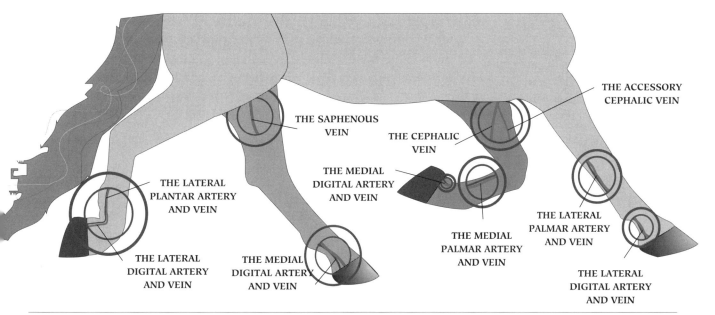

THE ACCESSORY CEPHALIC VEIN

THE SAPHENOUS VEIN

THE CEPHALIC VEIN

THE MEDIAL DIGITAL ARTERY AND VEIN

THE LATERAL PLANTAR ARTERY AND VEIN

THE MEDIAL PALMAR ARTERY AND VEIN

THE LATERAL PALMAR ARTERY AND VEIN

THE LATERAL DIGITAL ARTERY AND VEIN

THE MEDIAL DIGITAL ARTERY AND VEIN

THE LATERAL DIGITAL ARTERY AND VEIN

It's important that you understand what the bandage is being asked to do in this case. In the ideal, when immediate veterinary assistance is available, healing with a minimum of scar tissue is achieved by stitching the edges of the damaged tissues into proper position. This is not an option for your situation, so you must try to imitate the effect of stitches with your bandage.

So the bandage, besides keeping the wounded tissues protected and clean and absorbing exudates that ooze from them, should hold those tissues firmly in their proper positions so they'll knit together and anchor down to underlying tissues where they belong. The unstitched, unbandaged wound on a horse's leg almost always gapes open when the leg bears weight — you must try to prevent that, because the more the damaged tissues move and distort from their rightful position, the more scar tissue will be heaped onto the mess to try and stabilize it, and the bigger and lumpier the scar will be when it's all healed.

Therefore, by pressing the tissues into their proper positions, your bandage must counteract the effects of gravity, prevent or reduce edema and swelling that push them out of position from the inside, and support and limit movement of the leg so the tissues aren't tugged out of position by flexing joints and stretching skin. Furthermore, the bandage must not shift or bunch or otherwise apply uneven

STEP 12.
Bandage

SPECIAL NOTE 7.9

The woven gauze sponge is better than a non-stick pad for most superficial wounds because it will stick to the surface of the injured tissues and, when removed, pull a thin layer of mostly contaminated tissue off, leaving a cleaner surface (this is called debridement).

Sharp edges of metal buildings are the most common cause of lacerations like this one.

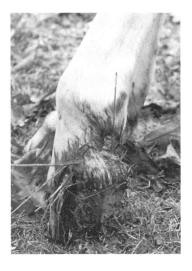

Try to stick to water-soluble dressings for use directly on wounds. Read the label for the words "in a water soluble base."

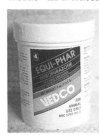

If it says "water removable," it's not water soluble.

pressure that might cause further tissue damage.

Another important function of the bandage is to eliminate "dead space" — a pocket that is created when tissue is pulled away from its underlying bed. Serum and debris can accumulate in this pocket and become infected. Your bandage should press these disrupted tissues against their underlying neighbors to eliminate the pocket until they become knitted together, but it must do this without interfering with circulation.

Whether your bandaging job is a breeze or a tough assignment will depend on the location of the injury. If it's in the vicinity of a joint, where there's necessarily a lot of movement, you've got a real challenge on your hands, and your prowess in skillful application of bandages is going to be tested. Depending on the bandaging materials available to you, choose and adapt a bandaging technique that will most closely provide the type of immobilization you'll need for your horse.

For a step-by-step description of some useful emergency bandages, along with instructions on how to apply, see *Chapter 18*.

SPECIAL NOTE 7.10

PHENYLBUTAZONE DOSAGE RECOMMENDATION FOR ANTIINFLAMMATORY TREATMENT IN SEVERE LACERATIONS:

800-1,000 lb horse:	1 gram
1,000-1,200 lb horse:	1-1/2 grams
1,200-1,400 lb horse:	2 grams

To be given orally, once only.

SPECIAL NOTE 7.11

BANAMINE™ DOSAGE RECOMMENDATION FOR ANTIINFLAMMATORY TREATMENT IN SEVERE LACERATIONS:

800-1,000 lb horse:	2 cc
1,000-1,200 lb horse:	3 cc
1,200-1,400 lb horse:	4 cc

To be given intramuscularly, once only.

Scrapes and Bruises

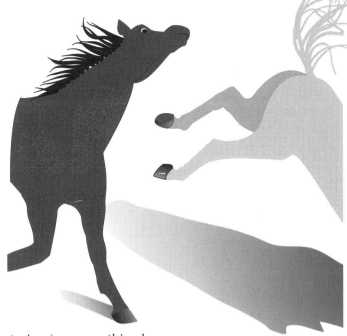

Most scrapes (abrasions) and bruises (contusions) are something less than emergencies — they're minor inconveniences, traditional "treatment" for the former being a dollop of antibiotic goo or an aerosol spritz of purple stuff, traditional treatment for the latter being "therapeutic neglect." But a scrape can be as serious as a third-degree burn if it's deep enough or covers a large enough area, and the damage from bruising, often underestimated because it's hidden under the skin, can be severe enough to threaten loss of function. With an understanding of what's happening inside with these injuries, you can take proper steps to minimize the damage they can do and help healing take place as quickly, and with as little scarring, as possible.

Abrasions

Abrasions (scrapes that remove superficial layers of skin or mucous membrane) are usually minor injuries unless they involve a large area, as might be the case when a horse falls out of a moving horse trailer onto a paved road, or falls while self-motivating at high speeds, or side-swipes a rough-surfaced obstacle.

What you see

Depending on the abrading surface (gravel, dirt, turf, asphalt, wood, etc.), abrasion injuries have the potential for entrenched contamination that must be removed for the skin to heal without complications such as infection, scarring, and proud flesh.

SPECIAL NOTE 8.1

It takes three to six hours for bacteria on the surface of a wound to penetrate deeper into the tissues in search of a place to create an infection. Once they've migrated beneath the surface, you can't get at them without removing live tissue. The moral of the story: clean that wound right away!

The best fluid for flushing wounds is sterile saline solution, the kind used for intravenous use (it's called "normal" saline, because its 0.9% strength is the same as normal serum). A good alternative is to make your own saline solution — it won't be sterile, but it'll be clean enough for most abrasions. Mix 4 tsp table salt in a gallon of clean, cool water (or 1 tsp per quart), and use this as your stock solution to refill your squirt bottle as needed.

What's going on inside

Many of the tiny blood vessels that nourish the skin have likely been damaged, resulting in slow oozing of blood from deeper tissues. Damaged nerve endings are firing, causing a stinging kind of pain. Serum, the liquid portion of blood, is seeping from damaged soft tissues. Undamaged blood vessels are dilating, opening tiny windows called *fenestrations* within their walls, to allow specialized white blood cells into the area to begin cleaning up the debris. Inflammation (seen as heat, swelling, redness, and pain), which is a natural and necessary part of the healing process, begins almost immediately, and the speed and severity with which it appears is directly related to the magnitude and depth of the abrasions — the more severe the injury, the faster the area swells and becomes hot and swollen. As the tissues swell, foreign material that was ground into the injured area becomes more deeply embedded.

Why is this injury dangerous?

It's rarely dangerous in the sense of life and death. But if an exceptionally broad area (25% or more of the horse's body) is involved in the abrasion, a significant volume of tissue fluid will be lost to oozing and seepage, leaving the animal vulnerable to infection and dehydration. The skin is an important first line of defense against microorganisms, and if enough of that skin has been damaged by this injury, the horse's immune status is just as jeopardized as it would have been if the same amount of his surface area had been burned.

But in most cases, the impending danger in an abrasion injury is cosmetic. If improperly managed, abrasions can become infected, which will delay healing and result in excessive scarring. And if the abrasion is located on the lower legs, proud flesh is also a possibility.

What would the vet do?

Most abrasions result in the "sanding away" of skin, leaving nothing to suture. Therefore, the primary treatment for abrasions is to clean them. Hydrotherapy (irrigating with water or, preferably, a mild salt [saline] solution) is the most effective way, using such basic instrumentation as a trigger-type spray bottle, a Water-Pik, or a garden hose, depending on the extent of the wound and how prepared the vet is. Bits of foreign material that are too deeply embedded to be dislodged by hydrotherapy are manually removed, and any tags or shreds of tissue that are likely devitalized are snipped off. If necessary, a sedative/painkiller is given to facilitate this process, but it's rarely necessary.

Depending on personal preference, the extent and location of the wound, and whether or not the immediate environment is likely to contaminate or irritate it (e.g., if the surroundings and time of year provide for dust, or pollen, or flies, or grass seeds, etc.), the vet might decide to apply a topical medication. Medication to be applied directly to the wound must not be irritating, and it should be water-soluble, rather than petrolatum-based. But normal skin, adjacent to the wound, is best protected with a light coating of a petrolatum-based antimicrobial ointment, because the serum and exudate that will leak from the wounds is an ideal medium for bacterial growth, and if allowed to build up and encrust on normal skin, it can create a nasty dermatitis. If the location and nature of the abrasion is such that bandaging is desired (for example, if it's on a lower limb and therefore prone to contamination and the formation of proud flesh), a lightweight Class II bandage is applied (see *Chapter 18*). Abrasion wounds in difficult-to-bandage locations (elbow, stifle, groin) might be treated instead with cyanoacrylate spray, a sort of aerosol "glue-bandage."

Systemic antimicrobial medication (pills, injections) are rarely indicated with abrasion wounds unless, again, the area abraded is exceptionally large and the vet is concerned that the horse is in danger of becoming systemically ill from absorbing microorganisms through the exposed raw tissues.

The horse's tetanus immunization status is checked and updated as needed — if a tetanus toxoid booster was given within the past six months, no additional booster is warranted. If it's been six to twelve months since the last booster, another booster is given. If it's been over 12 months or if the horse's tetanus immunization status is unknown, a tetanus *antitoxin* injection is given, and the vet may opt to give a separate injection of tetanus toxoid, in a separate site.

All abraded surfaces will ooze, ooze, ooze for the next three to seven days, so the vet will recommend that you clean away all the accumulated crust and debris every day to prevent bacterial infections that like to become established beneath the crust and delay or otherwise complicate healing.

There's no vet. What should you do?

Walk the horse to a well-drained area that won't become a quagmire if you get it wet. Minimal restraint should be needed.

The wound must be irrigated, preferably with a mild salt solution (see *Special Note 8.2*), although plain water is a good second choice. Use a trigger-type spray bottle, a 60-cc syringe with blunted needle, or a hose, in decreasing order of preference (but any of these choices is acceptable). Irrigate all abraded areas, starting with a slow trickle at the lower end of the wound, gradually working upward and building the water pressure to a medium spray. The goals are

1. to dissolve and wash away the natural film of viscous serum that has already congealed on the surface,

2. to overwhelm the firing nerve endings so they'll stop pin-pricking the horse (much the way your body becomes accustomed to what is initially a too-hot bath),

SPECIAL NOTE 8.3

On the unbandaged wound, flies can be a big problem — for them, serum and blood and pus are homing beacons, and they'll contaminate a wound with their filthy little fly feet, possibly even lay eggs in the disturbed tissues. The best fly control is cleanliness, both locally at the wound site and environmentally. Keep manure and urine-soaked bedding picked up and carried well away, and de-stink the area with a powdered stall refresher such as sweet PDZ™ or a spray solution of vinegar and water to keep flies from buzzing in to check out the ammonia smell common in areas chronically soaked with urine. A vigorous cleaning of the wound from one to three times daily , gently patting dry with a thick, clean towel, helps discourage them.

STEP 1.

Choose treatment area

STEP 2.

Flush the wound

SPECIAL NOTE 8.4

Try to stick to water-soluble dressings for use directly on wounds. Read the label for the words, "in a water soluble base." If it says, "water removable," it's not water soluble.

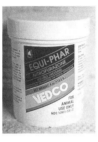

and

3. to dislodge and flush away any foreign material and bacteria that are stuck to the gooey exudate, blood, serum, and vulnerable soft tissues.

Bacteria adhere to the wound by an electrostatic charge that requires a light bombardment with your hose or spray bottle to shake them loose — dabbing a wound "clean" with a wet cloth merely pats the bacteria on their little heads and is totally ineffective in getting them off the wound.

All abraded areas should get about 15 minutes of this "hydrotherapy" for maximum benefit. Inspect closely for any deeply embedded foreign material that stubbornly remains afterwards and remove it with a clean gauze 4x4 sponge or clean, disinfected or sterilized tweezers.

STEP 3.
Dry, then medicate

If possible, allow the hosed area to air-dry so the oozing blood vessels, left undisturbed for several minutes, will have a chance to seal closed and clot. If conditions aren't conducive to air-drying, use a *clean* terrycloth towel or *clean* cotton cloth to dry the uninjured area around the wound, then use *clean*, brand new stacks of gauze 4 x 4 sponges to press and dab the wound dry (don't rub — you'll re-awaken broken blood vessels and get the blood oozing faster).

With a very clean finger, apply a thin film of water-based triple antibiotic cream (see *Special Note 8.4*) to all damaged tissues .

Then apply a petrolatum-based ointment to the normal skin surrounding the injured area, making the lower margins nice and wide to serve as a "drain board" for the serum and exudate that will ooze from the injured tissues.

STEP 4.
Tetanus

Check the horse's tetanus immunization status. If a tetanus toxoid booster was given within the past six months, no additional booster is warranted. If it's been 6 - 12 months since the last booster, give another. If it's been over 12 months or if the horse's tetanus immunization status is unknown, give a tetanus *antitoxin* injection, and give the toxoid in two weeks (see *Special Note 8.5* for the risks of using tetanus antitoxin). Mark your calendar so you don't forget.

STEP 5.
Bandage

Most researchers agree that wounds heal better if left open to the air, but in your case a bandage might be warranted to protect it from trauma (from walking through grass and brush, for example), to keep flies away, and to keep the area from swelling — it all depends on where the wound is and what your circumstances are. Choose a lightweight or medium weight Type II bandage (see *Chapter 18*) with an antibiotic ointment-coated gauze sponge directly against the lesion.

The accumulated crust, scale, and debris should be pummelled off daily with an initially gentle, eventually moderate stream of water from the hose every 8-24 hours for the next 3-4 days minimum, patting the lesion dry and rebandaging as needed to keep the tissues protected.

STEP 6.
Follow-up

SPECIAL NOTE 8.5

In rare instances, horses given tetanus antitoxin can develop a condition called "serum sickness" — they react to the proteins in the antitoxin and, months later, succumb to serious, often fatal, liver disease. All the more reason to keep your horse's tetanus vaccination status up-to-date so you can give a toxoid booster, rather than antitoxin, in the event of an injury.

Contusions

There is a tendency to minimize the destructive potential of bruises because they're not as ugly to look at as an open, gaping wound. However, injury from blunt trauma can be 100 times *more* likely to result in massive tissue destruction, necrosis, infection, and loss of function than a deep slicing wound because the force of the blunt trauma is usually exerted over a wider area, meaning that more total tissue is damaged, and blood vessels bringing vital nourishment to adjacent tissues are often crushed, leading to massive tissue death in areas that weren't even involved in the initial collision. Furthermore, the whole mess is hidden under the skin where dead tissue and blood can simply pool and decompose, providing an ideal life-support environment for bacteria anxious to play house inside your horse's damaged tissues.

Injury from blunt trauma can be 100 times more likely than a deep slicing laceration to cause massive tissue destruction.

What's going on inside?

When it's soft tissue only that has been traumatized, then at the very least, blood vessels have been broken, resulting in bleeding.

IF: the tissues in the damaged area are accommodating and loose, blood can accumulate, stretching out those tissues like a pelican sac.

IF: the tissues in the damaged area are tight and unable to stretch to accommodate accumulating blood, but the tissues *below* the damaged area are more stretchy, the blood can yield to gravity, spill between planes of muscle and sinew into the potential sacs below, and create a bizarre looking "goiter" full of blood.

IF: the tissues in the damaged area are tight and there's just nowhere for blood to go, the pressure in that area will act as a natural compression bandage and stop the flow of blood early, avoiding the formation of a blood "pocket."

When it's a bone that's been traumatized but no fracture occurred, then the periosteum (the Saran-Wrap-like coating over the bone) has been damaged — the equivalent of a "bruised shin" — and lameness will develop gradually as inflammation in the periosteum increases and brings an associated increase in heat, swelling, and pain. But if the injury caused major disruption of deep tissues (such as bone fracture or severance of a tendon), the lameness will appear immediately, and with one or two "test steps" the horse will quickly become "three-legged."

Why is this injury dangerous?

It's a gamble. A horse can absorb a terrific kick and suffer no significant consequences, while a lesser kick can be devastating — it all depends on the physics of the blow (the angle, the force, where it landed, etc.) Blunt trauma to the major muscle masses at the rump and/or upper rear leg, despite the bone-protective benefit of muscle padding, can be dangerous because of the risk of a condition called *compartmental syndrome* (see *Special Note 8.7*). Blunt trauma to the shoulder and/or upper foreleg threaten the "shoulder blade" (scapula), the shoulder joint itself, and a major nerve (the suprascapular nerve) that is briefly exposed as it emerges from beneath the scapula to run down the upper leg (direct damage to that nerve can literally ruin a foreleg). Dislocation of the shoulder joint is accompanied by massive destruction of muscle normally holding the joint together. Lower leg injuries can be dangerous because of the relative lack of protection to major supporting structures such as bone, tendon, blood vessel and ligament. And of course a blow to the head is in a category all its own. (For more on head trauma, see *Chapter 9*.)

SPECIAL NOTE 8.7

COMPARTMENTAL SYNDROME

The massive "meat" and sinew of the thick, upper legs are organized into six compartments, each compartment individually "wrapped" in a Saran-Wrap-like membrane called fascia. Major nerves and blood vessels run between the compartments like garden hoses nestled between mattresses. If the well-perfused muscle tissue of the leg is damaged, it'll bleed and swell like crazy, and all that loose fluid (blood and edema) within the muscle will begin to fill up the Saran-Wrap sleeve housing that particular compartment. In compartmental syndrome, that increased pressure impinges upon the major nerves and blood vessels coursing in the deep fascia between the compartments and causes signs ranging from mild soreness to complete anesthesia, paralysis, and Volkman's contracture (a deep "dimple" where muscle and/or tendon tissue died from lack of blood supply). The resultant impairment of circulation can permanently damage the affected limb, both in terms of its cosmetic appearance and its ability to function properly.

What would the vet do?

The vet's main advantage is the technology and know-how needed to get a definitive diagnosis — nerve blocks, x-ray, ultrasound, thermography, and/or nuclear scintigraphy (if associated with a big-bucks university), along with a skilled, experienced eye and hands-on examination, can spell the diagnosis out in black-and-white. To protect an injured leg from further damage while further diagnostic procedures are done, the vet can immobilize it with a rigid cast that the x-ray beam can "see" through. And, if necessary for diagnosis or treatment, the horse can be gently laid down with general anesthesia, preventing the usual crash by strapping the awake, standing horse to a vertical table, using the straps to support the slumping horse during induction, and then rotating the hydraulic table to the horizontal position and rolling it to the x-ray room. (Mobile vets, of course, won't have this kind of equipment, nor will they have a portable x-ray machine powerful enough to get decent x-rays of anything other than the lower parts of the leg.) Ultrasound examination will yield more information than x-rays if the injury is confined to soft tissues rather than bone.

If there's a fracture, various options to immobilize the fracture are available, depending on what bone is involved and what sort of architecture the fracture presents. There are a lot of variables that must be considered in determining the treatment, including your finances. Treatment options might include stall rest, splinting, casting, surgery, or a combination of the above — the techniques available are as varied as the injuries, and it's no longer assumed that a horse with a fracture should be put to sleep.

There's no vet. What should you do?

FOR BLUNT TRAUMA TO THE LOWER LEG:

In injuries to the lower leg, you might have a tough time deciding how bad it is on the inside — is it just a badly bruised shin, or could it be something so severe as a cracked bone or a lacerated tendon? Until you have the answer to that question, the best thing to do, especially if your horse is severely lame, is to immobilize the leg until you can get him to an equipped equine veterinary hostpital for a definitive diagnosis. Assume the worst and hope for the best. Your goals are:

1. to arrest the hemorrhage and swelling and

2. to prevent further damage from distortion of the injured tissues. You accomplish these goals by wrapping the leg in a compression-type bandage and by "freezing" the leg in a position that permits the horse to balance but prevents the inner parts of the leg from moving.

STEP 1.
Ice the injured leg

Ice the leg while you're gathering supplies for bandaging and splinting. Don't move the horse or ask him to bear weight on the injured leg — bring your supplies to him where he stands. Icing techniques include

a. plunging the leg into a bucket of ice water for five minutes at a time, every 20 minutes, for 1 hour (or until the leg is appropriately bandaged and splinted, whichever happens first), or

b. wrapping packs of crushed ice, bags of frozen peas or corn, or chemical cool-packs directly onto the leg with a track wrap.

STEP 2.
Apply a compression bandage

The compression bandage will gently but firmly apply pressure to the soft tissues to help stop any ongoing bleeding and to prevent edema from the inflammation that is building around the injury. A heavyweight Type III bandage would be warranted for a severe injury (see *Chapter 18*).

STEP 3.
Apply a splint, if and only if...

Apply a field splint over the bandage to make it rigid so the leg can't bend the joints above and below the injury. This means the splint must extend *above* the joint that is above the injury and it must extend *below* the joint that is below the injury. If you can't accomplish this, don't apply a splint at all — instead of immobilizing the leg, it can potentially *cause* damaging movement of the internal parts.

There are several splints that are feasible for field use. See *Chapter 18* for help in deciding which to use.

STEP 4.
Support the other legs

Apply heavyweight Type III-IV partial-support bandages to the other three lower legs for support (see *Special Note 8.8*), since they're now carrying the load of four legs.

SPECIAL NOTE 8.8

If the leg needs to be splinted, apply a *splint*. Don't be misled by the term "support bandage." Research has shown that so-called support bandages, which usually consist of substantial elastic wraps applied to the leg under considerable tension, are very effective in reducing swelling, but they do not relieve strain on the leg's supportive structures. In a study comparing the support given by a rigid cast, a splint, and a support bandage, the strain on the suspensory apparatus of the leg (the suspensory ligament, the deep digital flexor tendon, and the superficial digital flexor tendon) was reduced by 67%, 30% and 0%, respectively.

The support bandage can be a useful underlayer, but in order to alleviate stress on the leg, the wrap must be made rigid by additional external means (see *Chapter 18*).

Give no painkillers or antiinflammatories. Until the extent of the problem has been diagnosed, any drugs that might make the horse more comfortable might encourage him to over-use the leg.

STEP 5.
Give no drugs.

Get to the nearest competent equine veterinarian without delay.

STEP 6.
Hit the road

FOR BLUNT TRAUMA TO HEAVILY MUSCLED AREAS SUCH AS UPPER LEG, SHOULDER, OR BRISKET:

The main aim in treating injuries involving heavily muscled areas is to get the internal bleeding stopped as soon as possible so as to minimize the final size of the bruise and to keep the area of damaged tissue as small as possible. This is best done by

1. restricting muscle movement (so that torn intramuscular blood vessels have a chance to seal over),

2. lowering the blood pressure (to slow down the hemorrhage), and

3. applying cold compression (to slow blood supply to the damaged area, and to slow the metabolism of adjacent tissues, thereby decreasing their immediate needs for blood and increasing the odds that they'll survive the interruption in their blood supply).

Do not move the horse—treat him where he stands, and confine him there for at least two hours before slowly moving him, if necessary, to a stall or other enclosure.

STEP 1.
FREEZE!

Apply packs of crushed ice or chemical cold packs that are large and/or numerous enough to chill adjacent, uninjured tissue as well as the entire injured area. Hold them in place with firmly applied track wraps or, if the area does not lend itself to bandaging, manually press and hold the packs directly over the point of impact for 20 minutes, then off for ten minutes, then back on for 20 minutes, until two hours have passed.

STEP 2.
Ice the injured area

While someone else is pressing the ice packs in place with firm, consistent pressure, lower the horse's blood pressure with one of the non-medical techniques detailed on pages 124–125. Strive to achieve profound relaxation, which the horse will signify by sighing deeply, lowering his head, and chewing absent-mindedly.

STEP 3.
Calm the horse.

After at least two hours of immobility, calming, and ice pack-pressure, slowly and quietly walk the horse to prevent stiffening.

STEP 4.
Hand-walk

Should you seek veterinary assistance?

Yes, if you have any reason to believe that there has been significant internal damage. The vet might discover that in order to prevent compartmental syndrome, the accumulated blood and serum will need to be drained out. If a section of tissue has died because of the injury, the dead tissue will do what you'd expect: it'll rot. To prevent abscessation and infection of adjacent, healthy tissues, surgery might be required to remove the dead tissue.

Injury to the Face and Head

Superficial head/face wounds
Facial bone fractures
Brain trauma

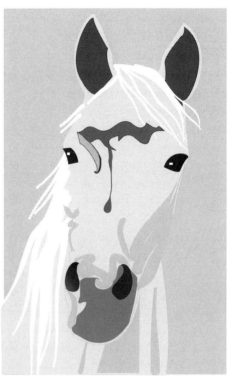

The most important thing to remember about a head wound in a horse, assuming the brain is uninjured, is that it probably isn't as horrible as it looks. Even the most gruesome wounds on the head usually heal beautifully, and even if you're initially dissatisfied with the way a head wound heals, don't despair — Mother Nature is a slow but accomplished plastic surgeon, and many head wounds continue to reshape and remodel months and even years after the original injury. And if you're in a hurry for results, head wounds generally respond very well to plastic surgery done by humbler veterinary surgeons. Unlike certain other areas of the body, such as the legs, heads are cheerful cooperators that tolerate natural and artificial remodeling procedures without the pesky tendency to overreact (i.e., proud flesh). So, with some important exceptions, the head is one of the "best" places for an injury.

What you see

Blood, blood, blood. Blood coming from the wound, maybe even from one or both nostrils. The circulation to the soft tissues of the face and head is exuberant, and at no time is this more obvious than when an injury occurs. Since many of these injuries occur when a curious horse carefully sticks his head where it doesn't belong, then violently yanks it back out when he encounters a problem, it's common for him to catch a wrinkle on, for example, a protruding nailhead and pull up a triangle of skin.

If the injury has fractured any of the bones of the face, you might also see gross distortion, such as a "caved-in" area.

What does bleeding from the nostrils mean? *In the case of trauma-associated nosebleed, it's probably just a few broken blood vessels high in the nasal cavity, but if it's severe it could spell much more serious injury at the back of the throat or at the base of the brain. The only way to know for sure is to have the horse examined endoscopically ("scoped").*

Deeper injuries, involving trauma to the brain, will yield a spectrum of signs from temporary confusion and dizziness to permanent blindness, convulsions, coma, and death.

Why are head wounds dangerous?

Most head injuries in horses are surface wounds that disrupt the cushion of soft tissues outside the skull or, in more severe cases, fracture the bones of the face. In such cases, the main danger is cosmetic, although sometimes the functioning of an injured part, such as an eyelid, a sinus, a nostril, or a lip, is impaired.

But without a doubt, the most dangerous head wound is the one that threatens the integrity of the brain. Any head wound that results from a collision of any sort — horse with horse, horse with tree, horse with car, horse with overhead beam, horse with ground (as in horse flips over and lands on head)— risks brain trauma and its accompanying potential for intracranial bleeding and/or swelling.

Most brain injuries in horses are the result of inertia, the law of physics that states that moving objects tend to want to continue moving at the same speed and in the same direction, and objects that are motionless tend to want to stay put. Like a Fabergé egg packed in a shipping crate with not quite enough packing material, the brain can injure itself by smashing into the walls of the crate (skull) meant to protect it. If a horse runs headlong into a tree, for example (it isn't as rare as you might think), the impact of the head with the tree may not be nearly as devastating as the impact of the brain with the inside of the skull when the forces of inertia carry it forward into that unyielding wall of bone.

What's going on inside?

How can a bump on the head cause blindness? *A blow to the back of the head will jog the brain backward, toward the back of the skull. This puts a tug on the optic nerve — the "cable" that connects the eyeball to the brain — and can functionally sever that connection. The affected eye might look normal, but it sees nothing.*

In the case of the **surface head wound**, three things are happening:

1. Flaps of tissue are drying, curling, and shrinking, which will make it more difficult to piece them back into their original positions.

2. The longer those flaps remain separated from their usual blood supply, dangling and drying and becoming contaminated in the cruel air, the worse are their chances of surviving to see a suture needle.

3. Injured tissues with intact blood supply are becoming inflamed: increasingly hot, swollen, and painful with each passing minute. As a result, separations in the skin are widening as the tissue swells, tightens, and pulls apart.

In the case of **facial bone fracture**, there might be only a crack without displacement, or the broken area of bone might be pushed inward. If any fragments of bone are protruding through the skin, they were probably levered to their outward position by their opposite ends being pushed inward.

In the case of **brain trauma**, often (but not always) accompanied by fracture of facial bones and/or skull, the brain tissue reacts similarly to any other traumatized tissue: it becomes inflamed, which means swelling. Trouble is, there's no room for swelling within the confines of the skull, and if the trauma was severe enough, sufficient swelling will occur to cause a significant increase in pressure. The outward symptoms of brain trauma are, as a result, somewhat delayed — the impairment of the brain comes on gradually as the swelling and, therefore, the pressure, increase. If that pressure isn't arrested and relieved soon, *permanent* damage will occur to the delicate, irreplaceable cells of the brain.

The effects are the same if, instead of swelling, the brain is bleeding. If any of the delicate blood vessels in or around the brain was torn when the brain was jostled, the blood leaking into the cramped cranial quarters will create pressure on tissues that simply can't tolerate pressure, and a gradual derangement of function will be the result.

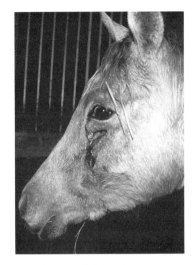

Facial wounds like this one can heal beautifully with little or no scar.

What would the vet do?

If a brisk assessment of the horse's pupils and gross reflexes, plus witnesses' accounts of what happened, confirm that the brain is likely to have been traumatized, the sharp veterinarian will immediately administer medications to lower the blood pressure, arrest or at least slow any intracranial bleeding, soothe traumatized tissues into postponing the inflammatory response they'd planned, and reduce any inflammation that has already started. With experience in head trauma cases, vets learn to turn a blind eye to any surface head wounds, no matter how gruesome they may be, until all possible steps have been taken to minimize the consequences of the injury to the brain.

Head-injured horses trailered to university veterinary hospitals for immediate reconstructive surgery on their fractured faces have been known to walk into the hospital, take their anesthetic normally, sleep well through their surgeries, and never wake up from anesthesia because of ongoing brain swelling and bleeding, magnified thanks to the additional trauma of the trip and the treatment. Furthermore, there's a narrow window of opportunity to get those "brain treatments" accomplished — once symptoms of brain injury begin to appear, they tend to escalate quickly, and the swelling and hemorrhage, and the associated damage to brain cells, get farther and farther along until they're out of reach of all medical efforts to reverse them. Reconstructive efforts to the surface wounds can wait.

If there is no reason to believe the brain has been traumatized, the vet will probably administer one of the popular alpha-2-agonist-class equine sedatives (xylazine or detomidine) that give threefold benefits: they sedate, they lower the head, and they provide some pain relief. If necessary, the injured tissues are also

SPECIAL NOTE 9.1

Is he brain-injured? The most important sign of brain injury is staying down for more than 4 hours after the trauma, or lying down soon afterward and staying down, and acting "dull," as though in a stupor. A head-trauma case that gets up but then lies down again may be experiencing inflammation or hemorrhage in the brain.

"numbed" with local anesthetic. General anesthesia is rarely needed for treatment of surface head wounds. The nicely sedated, nerve-blocked head is then meticulously cleaned, trimmed, and stitched together, and a bandage of some sort might be applied to press the injured tissues into position, prevent swelling from developing and tugging at the stitches, and to prevent the horse from rubbing at itchy, healing wounds and inadvertently ripping the whole thing open again.

There's no vet. What should you do?

STEP 1.
Calm the horse

It sounds impossible, but try to remain calm, and try to exude calmness to your horse. High blood pressure and its associated bleeding and swelling, whether inside or outside the skull, will only continue if the horse senses anxiety and panic from you.

STEP 2.
Look for signs of fracture

Gently explore the wounds with the fleshy part of your clean fingertips, feeling for crepitus — the popply, effervescent feeling (like beer in a Baggie) that signals possible bone fracture. If you feel crepitus, stop right there — don't keep exploring for the actual fracture, because your digital intrusion can stir up already damaged tissues.

STEP 3a.
If no fracture, apply ice and pressure

If you found no crepitus, and you have no reason to believe there are any fractures of the facial bones, then apply ice packs and moderate pressure directly over the wounds. A half-gallon plastic freezer bag with about a quart of crushed ice in it, laid over a clean dishtowel (to cushion the skin from sharp ice edges) and held with gentle, firm hand pressure is a good start until you get organized — it's important to get the ice on quickly. When your "go-fer" brings you more supplies, you can replace hand pressure with a track wrap or two, securing the ice bag in place with figure-eight passes of the wrap, using one or both ears as anchors and being careful not to strangle the horse by running tight wraps over the throat.

STEP 3b.
Unsure? Apply ice without pressure

If, on the other hand, you did feel crepitus, apply the ice without pressure so you don't risk compressing a shard of fractured bone into underlying tissue.

STEP 4a.
Clean the wound

If you don't suspect any bony fractures, inspect the surface wounds after 20 minutes of ice treatment. Flush them gently with a mild salt solution (see *Special Note 9.2*) made with lukewarm water — cold water would, technically, be better for the wound, but the horse is more likely to react to cold water by jerking his head up and deciding that you will get no further access. If your horse tolerates the twitch well, you might want to apply it now, for the endorphins it will release from the brain (natural morphine-like chemicals that calm the horse and numb his pain). If he doesn't tolerate the twitch, or if you're not sure of how he'll react to it, don't risk a fracas. Instead, just be patient and slow, and try to let your finesse substitute for more extreme restraint measures.

If, on the other hand, you do suspect bony fractures, simply do the best you can to gently pick out any obvious debris that is contaminating the wound. If you get any more involved than that, you risk disturbing the fracture site.

Cover the wound with a soft, very clean pad liberally coated with a completely water-soluble antibiotic dressing. A good choice for the pad would be a disposable diaper, trimmed to fit the horse, or a thick Kotex™ pad. If gauze 4 x 4 squares are all you have, apply several stacks adjacent to each other to cover the entire wound. Secure the padding in place with a roll or two of stretch gauze or a soft track wrap, making figure-eights that go in front, then in back, of an ear, and bridging the lower jaw bones rather than "throttling" the horse at the neck. For added bandage security, you can gently "dress" the head in a "queen-size" nylon stocking. Cut the foot off first, roll the leg up, and slip the roll over the horse's muzzle. Then slowly unroll it, carefully cutting holes for the eyes and ears. If it's too tight around the upper part of the horse's head, you can slit the stocking under the jaw. If the wound is near an eye, it might be easier to simply cover that eye with the dressing, making it stay closed, rather than try to keep the bandage's edges from creeping up and irritating the open eye. Whenever possible, utilize an ear to help anchor a head dressing, making sure the base of the ear is not being pinched. After the bandage is completely applied and taped, put the halter on over the whole thing. For more on head dressings, see *Chapter 18*.

STEP 5.
Dress the wound

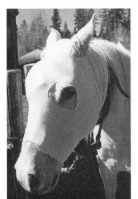 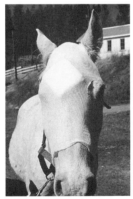

A stockinette or a leg from a men's large longjohns makes a good bandage for holding a stack of gauze over a facial wound. It can be secured with a stretchy adhesive tape (Expandover™ is especially suited for this), and with the halter on over the bandage, the horse is unlikely to disturb it. See *Chapter 18*.

SPECIAL NOTE 9.3

DOSAGE RECOMMENDATION FOR BANAMINE IN SEVERE HEAD WOUNDS:	
800 lb horse:	4 cc
900 lb horse:	4-1/2 cc
1,000 lb horse:	5 cc
1,100 lb horse:	5-1/2 cc
1,200 lb horse:	6 cc
1,300 lb horse:	6-1/2 cc
1,400 lb horse:	7 cc

To be given intramuscularly, once only.

Whether or not brain trauma is suspected, it's logical to give an antiinflammatory medication at this point to help control any inflammation that will be developing in the damaged tissues. If you have a prescription for Banamine injectable, follow the dosage guidelines in *Special Note 9.3* unless you have specific instructions from your veterinarian to give less than the amount in the chart. Do not give aspirin, especially if you suspect brain trauma, because aspirin will "thin the blood" (slow down its ability to clot) and encourage bleeding in the brain.

STEP 6.
If your vet gave you a prescription of Banamine™, this is a good time to give it.

STEP 7.
Apply DMSO

SPECIAL NOTE 9.4

DMSO is not appropriate for most "fresh" wounds, but its special properties make it a good choice for head wounds when brain trauma is a possibility.

Because of its value in decreasing brain swelling, DMSO is often administered intravenously by emergency veterinarians and trauma room physicians when they're dealing with head-trauma patients. If you have any topical DMSO solution or gel, which is a potent antiinflammatory medication that is instantly absorbed through the skin and into the bloodstream, you can moisten a clean, water-dampened cloth with about a teaspoon of DMSO and swab it onto the front of the horse's neck. For optimal absorption, make sure it's mixed with water, either by using the aforementioned damp cloth or by swabbing it onto clean, wet skin. Wear gloves to avoid absorbing it through your own skin, and absolutely do not mix it with any other substances or swab it onto skin that already has any chemicals on it (such as hair conditioner or liniment or a leg blister) — the DMSO can "drag" toxic elements from the skin right into the bloodstream.

STEP 8.
Tetanus

Check tetanus immunization status and act accordingly: If a tetanus toxoid booster was given within the past six months, no additional booster is warranted. If it's been six to twelve months since the last booster, give another. If it's been over 12 months, or if the horse's tetanus immunization status is unknown, give a tetanus *antitoxin* injection, and give the toxoid in two weeks (see *Special Note 9.5* for the risks of using tetanus antitoxin).

> **SPECIAL NOTE 9.5**
>
> In rare instances, horses given tetanus antitoxin can develop a condition called "serum sickness" — they react to the proteins in the antitoxin and, months later, succumb to serious, often fatal, liver disease. All the more reason to keep your horse's tetanus vaccination status up-to-date so you can give a toxoid, rather than antitoxin, in the event of an injury.

STEP 9.
Observe quietly

If you have reason to suspect that brain trauma might have occurred, create a quiet, stimulus-free environment for the horse to spend the next 12 to 24 hours while you keep a close eye on his progress. Rather than moving him to a veterinary hospital and subjecting him to the stress of a trailer ride, try to find a good equine vet that will come to you. Every hour, have a seat where you can watch him for several minutes without disturbing him, then approach him calmly and quietly for a closer look as you try to assess the following, being sure to write down your observations.

1. How's his attitude? Depressed? In a daze? Anxious?
2. Are his pupils the same size? Are his eyes shifting rhythmically from side to side? Are any eyelids drooping? When he blinks, do both lids blink together, or is one side unable to blink?

3. Does he seem able to walk normally, or does he seem off balance, or very stiff, or unable or unwilling to move? Or does he only want to turn in a circle? Is his head tilted? Does he press it on the wall?

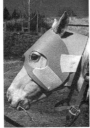 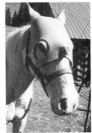

4. As you watch him and time ticks by, is he getting worse, or better, or staying the same?

5. Are parts of his face drooping, as though paralyzed? Can he control his tongue? Is either nostril pulled to one side?

6. Is he breathing normally, or is he breathing erratically?

If no brain trauma is suspected, it should be okay to head for home (if it's a minor injury or if you're within a half-day's drive) or for the nearest competent equine veterinarian's establishment (if the injury will require a closer look, possibly with sedation, and maybe some stitches).

If your horse seems unstable (wobbling or behaving strangely, for example), if he's had any convulsions, if he's in a coma, or if your hourly assessments suggest that his brain function is questionable and/or worsening, it's a good idea to protect his head from further damage in case he falls or thrashes. See *Special Note 9.6*.

How serious is his brain trauma?

Abnormalities in attitude, eyes, breathing patterns, posture and motor control can indicate injury to specific areas of the brain and brainstem and should be brought to the attention of the veterinarian as soon as he/she arrives — this will yield the beginnings of a prognosis. Actually, however, the horse's *progress* tells you more about his prospects than the specific symptoms tell you because no matter what area was injured, if it can recover from the injury your horse will be okay. In other words, if his condition is deteriorating before your eyes, odds are the internal damage is extensive and likely to be devastating. If, on the other hand, he shows evidence of possible brain damage, but his condition appears stable or, better yet, he seems to be improving, the damage is likely to be less extensive and *reversible*. In most cases, prompt and proper attention, refraining from radical treatment such as general anesthesia and surgery until a few days have passed, and keeping the environment calm and stimulus-free (avoiding a high-speed, bumpy, panic-stricken trailer ride) would be the approach that's in the best interest of the horse.

SPECIAL NOTE 9.6

A commercial crash helmet or a homemade protective hood (made with a dense, small-cell backpackers' mattress) can help protect the unstable or violent horse against further trauma to the head. See *Chapter 18* for more on how to make and apply a protective hood.

STEP 10.
Protect his head

SPECIAL NOTE 9.7

Don't try to assess your horse's eyesight. If his headache is severe enough, he may seem blind even though his eyesight is fine — vision is just an annoying chore when your head hurts. But if his brain has been injured, the horse's menace response may be exaggerated — instead of blinking or flinching when you put your hand in front of him, he might flip over backward.

SPECIAL CASE NOTES

Every head injury is different. Following are some points you should consider regarding specific types of head injury. If your horse's injury includes any of these features, be sure to read these notes.

SPECIAL CASE #1:
Injury to the tongue

Horses aren't linguists, and they use primarily their lips, rather than the tongue, to pick up food. Therefore, the tongue is an inessential structure, and if it's injured severely enough, amputation is always available as a last resort. Repairing a damaged tongue is usually rewarding, however, and the healing process is incredibly fast. The tissues of the inside of the mouth are accustomed to living fast, dying young and being replaced in a constant cycle of ongoing regeneration anyway, so there should be no trouble in repairing most types of wounds. Most tongue wounds that require surgery can be fixed with the horse awake, sedated, and with benefit of local anesthesia, although some surgeons prefer general anesthesia for some of the more severe cases. Untreated cuts of the tongue usually heal with no problems as far as the function of the tongue is concerned, although there is often some disfigurement. The main thing to remember about tongue wounds is to *look for them* so that if treatment is needed, it can be provided while the wound is still fresh.

SPECIAL CASE #2:
The lips and the teeth

Shallow wounds of the lips usually heal quickly and without significant scarring. Deep lip cuts, however, tend to heal with some bumps or dips that weren't there before, and surgical repair is needed to improve the outcome. Since many lip wounds are the result of a forced encounter of the lip with adjacent teeth, the teeth should always be examined for damage as well. Adult teeth that have been knocked out are often salvagable if the vet can replace them quickly, cleanly, and anchor them to adjacent teeth with wire (see *Special Note 9.8*). This almost always requires general anesthesia. Broken or displaced baby teeth, however, are usually just pulled out, since they have very short roots, a short natural lifespan, and they tend to get infected if left in place after being traumatically disrupted. Since the lips and the teeth are closely associated with the bones of the jaw, any injury to one of these structures should make examination of the others automatic.

SPECIAL CASE #3:
The eyelids

The eyelashes are very important to the eyes, so if an eyelid is damaged in any way, every effort should be made to save the edges that house the eyelashes and their follicles. As a rule, eyelid tissue survives and heals if given half a chance, so if an injury to an eyelid leaves a flap of eyelid tissue that looks "iffy," the experienced vet will still try to sew it back rather than remove it — this decision can always be changed later. New eyelashes will not grow if the follicles were removed with the flap. And if it looks like the flap of eyelid hanging over your horse's eye is too short, don't despair — the muscles within the eyelid tend to contract, making the flap curl up and appear too short to go back into place, but it'll stretch out again when the vet stitches it into place. If your horse's eyelid is lacerated, clean the wounded area gently with sterile eye-wash solution (it's a weak salt solution, but don't use the homemade stuff — for use around an eye it must be sterile). If you don't have eyewash solution, it's probably better to just pick out the "big pieces" of debris and skip the washing step. Cover the closed eye with a half-inch stack of clean gauze 4 x 4 squares onto which you've gobbed a mound of antibiotic ophthalmic ointment, and bandage the makeshift patch into place with a Type II or III head wrap (see *Chapter 18*) — this keeps it moist, helps to minimize bacterial growth, and protects it from further contamination and trauma. Even if the nearest vet is a long drive away, the laceration can be sutured the next day when you prepare it this way. This wrap also helps keep the eyeball moist. For more on eyelid injury, see *Chapter 11: The Troubled Eye*.

If an adult tooth has been completely dislodged, put it into a cup of milk while you wait for the vet — it'll be more likely to "take" if you store it this way.

If a trauma was severe enough to cause a fracture of the bones of the face, the odds are that the brain got bounced around as well. Unless there are extenuating circumstances, then, you should not be in too big a hurry to subject your traumatized horse to anesthesia and surgical repair of his broken facial bones. If there's a damaged cranial blood vessel on the verge of rupture, for example, the stress of anesthesia and a rocky recovery may be all that is required for that blood vessel to rupture and cause fatal brain hemorrhage. The fracture can wait until the horse's condition is stable, and in the meantime there are a lot of things you and a vet can be doing to stabilize the horse and improve the appearance and state of the injured tissues. A little time — perhaps as little as three days or so — should be sufficient for the damaged blood vessels to become fortified enough to withstand the stresses of surgery.

SPECIAL CASE #4:

The facial bones

Another consideration if facial bones are fractured is the sinuses — if the sinuses are involved in the fracture, they may be contaminated and may be in need of help to get cleaned out. Repair of a facial fracture will do little to help the horse's appearance if he begins to emit a foul odor and adopt a lop-sided appearance as his infected sinus festers, swells and eventually bursts. While repairing the fractured facial bones, the veterinarian will need to investigate the sinuses, and if necessary he/she can open them for drainage.

Damage to the facial nerve, which runs unprotected across the face, can affect the horse's ability to blink and make tears. This puts the eyeball at risk of drying out. Whenever the face has been traumatized, be sure to treat the eyes with ophthalmic ointment (your triple antibiotic ophthalmic ointment is fine) to lubricate them just in case. When you arrive at the vet's, he/she can evaluate the facial nerve.

Other evidence of facial nerve damage: a drooping ear, a drooping eyelid, drooping lips, or a nostril pulled toward the unaffected side.

The pinna (upright portion) of the ear is made like a cartilage sandwich — an ear-shaped piece of cartilage loosely sandwiched between two ear-shaped pieces of skin.

SPECIAL CASE #5:

The ears

An injury here can cause an accumulation of debris and fluids that fill up the pinna like a little pillow, and surgical drainage becomes necessary. If the cartilage becomes infected, you may be in for a long, chronic battle. Small wounds are probably best cleaned, trimmed as needed, and left unsutured. Larger wounds that require stitches are complicated by the fact that cartilage does not suture well, and stitching ears through the cartilage tends to encourage the formation of scar tissue which, by nature, tends to shrink as it matures. This can lead to puckers and "dogeared" margins of the affected ear.

SPECIAL CASE #6:
The horse that flipped over backward

Horses, especially youngsters, have a habit of rearing up during forceful halter training, ear clipping, trailer loading, tying, or tightening a girth. There are some specific injuries that are more common in the horse that flipped over backward, sustaining a blow to the back of the head, than in other types of head trauma.

The optic nerve — the "cable" that connects the eyeball to the brain — appears to be quite sensitive to any kind of disturbance, and when the back of the head is jarred, the brain is jolted backward, thereby tugging on the optic nerve. A horse in this situation might be immediately blind, or his blindness — in one or both eyes — might not be noticed for a few days. The vet will have to administer high-powered antiiflammatory medication to soothe the irritated nerve.

Another common injury under these circumstances is fracture of the *hyoid apparatus*. This is a sling, made of delicate bones, that supports the root of the tongue, the voicebox, and the back of the throat. When the horse flips over, the muscles at the front of the neck are tense, holding the chin toward the chest, and at the point of impact, the chin flies back, which flings the chin skyward, violently twangs the muscles and snaps the hyoid bone. The affected horse will have difficulty swallowing, and his tongue might protrude from his mouth. Any handling of the tongue and any attempts to open the mouth will be deeply resented — it's extremely painful. Obviously he can't eat this way — a veterinarian will have to feed him by stomach tube and/or intravenously until his injuries can be repaired.

When the point of impact in the flipping horse is the poll, the most common injury is fracture of the base of the skull. As with hyoid bone fractures, the skull base fracture is usually the result of neck muscles forcefully yanking on the bones when the head hits and the tucked chin is suddenly flung skyward from the force and inertia of the fall. Bleeding from the nose or ears, lack of balance, a tilting head, and walking in an endless circle are common signs. The horse is usually very unstable when trying to walk, and he may be particularly "spooky," so be very careful — put him in a quiet, stimulus-free place and be wary for your own safety when you're in there with him. Put his feed and water nearby so he doesn't have to move to get to them, and if possible have them anchored to the wall so he can't knock them down and panic. Again, find a vet who will come to you — don't trailer the horse, or you risk further trauma.

C H A P T E R   1 0

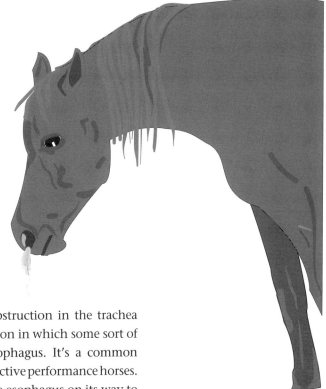

Choke

Some might think that "choke" refers to an obstruction in the trachea (windpipe) — but in horses, choke is a condition in which some sort of foreign mass has become lodged in the esophagus. It's a common problem in horses of all ages, but it's especially common in active performance horses. It's almost always due to a wad of feed getting stuck in the esophagus on its way to the stomach.

What you see

The choked horse will show a variety of symptoms, depending on how long the choke has existed.

FRESH CHOKE
(happened within the
past hour)

- drooling
- extending head and neck
- constant chewing, sometimes with lips distorted into a grimace
- repeatedly swallowing
- retching, as though trying to vomit

OLDER CHOKE
(happened more than an
hour ago)

- all of the fresh choke signs, plus:
- coughing
- regurgitation of saliva-mixed "pea soup" dripping from the nostrils
- frequent and loud snorting to clear the nostrils

For the most part, diagnosing choke is easy: any horse that is drooling and regurgitating (a greenish "pea soup" or chewed food slurry spilling from one or both nostrils) while showing no signs of colic is choked until proven otherwise.

However, there is one BIG exception: always bear in mind that regurgitation and drooling can also be signs of **rabies.** If you have any doubts, hands off. Get help. Period.

Wait a minute...

You thought only toothless old-timers choked? Think again. Your own horse is a prime choke candidate if he fits into any of the following scenes:

- He's choked before (it can happen to any horse, but some horses tend to do it over and over again during their lifetimes).

Always bear in mind that regurgitation and drooling can also be signs of RABIES.

- He was recently medicated with an oral bolus (a real "horse pill" — the pill is forced to the back of the horse's throat, usually using a barbaric device called a balling gun, which carries a very real risk of traumatizing the inside of the horse's mouth and throat. The pill itself, which usually has sharp edges and contains dry, irritating chalk-like ingredients, can easily get stuck sideways in the esophagus and sit there, ready to create a logjam the next time the horse eats).

- He recently had a different sort of problem in his neck: e.g., infection from an intramuscular injection in the neck, or a kick to the neck, or a recently botched intravenous injection of phenylbutazone ("bute") or the antibiotic drug trimethoprim-sulfamethoxazole/sulfadiazine (Tribrissen™), either of which can, if leakage occurs outside the vein into the tissues around it, cause a hotbed of inflammation that might possibly affect the esophagus.

- He's a piggy eater — he can't seem to eat fast enough to satisfy himself, or he's afraid that neighboring horses will steal his food, and he bolts whole mouthfuls without taking the time to chew and swallow before taking the next mouthful.

- He's got some weird eating habits, consuming such delicacies as fenceboards, or tree bark, or plastic bags, or toys, or sawdust bedding.

- He was recently treated with an oral paste medication — some, not all, of these medications can irritate and burn the mouth and esophagus, especially if the horse vigorously resists being medicated.

Horses that are anxious travelers are prone to choking

- He's a "poor traveler," exhibiting anxious or apprehensive behavior while being trailered. Some poor travelers will refuse to drink (or not have any water offered to them by neglectful handlers) and nervously grab and gobble hay, swallowing it without chewing — these horses are prime candidates for choke.

- He's aged, needs his teeth floated, or has any other condition that might affect his ability to adequately chew his food.

- He wears a halter all the time, and "for safety's sake" you make sure it's pretty snug (but you forgot that it might interfere with his ability to chew).

- A big part of his diet is pelleted food. Pellets are often implicated in chokes because they tend to swell up when wetted.

- He was recently given a "treat" of apple, apple core, or carrot which, if gobbled up and swallowed whole, could easily get stuck on the way down.

In many cases, however, the horse "just chokes" — there's no apparent rhyme or reason.

Frankly, most chokes resolve themselves — that's the good news. The bad news is, the longer a choke persists, the more the muscles around it will spasm or clench, grabbing the obstruction in an iron fist, "locking" the choke in place and setting up an escalating inflammation around it.

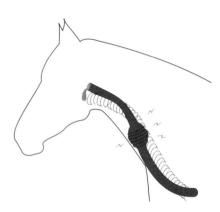

Why is choke dangerous?

When a horse chokes, five dangerous things can happen:

1. It's not uncommon for choked horses to continue eating and drinking, which causes regurgitation of a juicy, soupy slurry of chewed food, saliva, and water. Regurgitated food, which must come up the esophagus and out through the nose (the horse can't "vomit" in the usual sense), has a perfect opportunity to spill back down the windpipe and into the lungs where it can cause a raging pneumonia.

Where they begin at the throat, the esophagus lies above the opening to the windpipe. If the head is elevated, any regurgitation is likely to spill into the windpipe where it can roll down into the lungs and cause pneumonia. With the head down, regurgitated material spills out onto the ground instead.

2. The muscles of the esophagus become irritated by the prolonged presence of the obstruction — these muscles are accustomed to food passing through, but they're easily "annoyed" when a wad of food decides to hang around. They become inflamed, and they express their inflammation by clenching around the obstruction. This makes it less likely that the obstruction will resolve itself, and it becomes more likely that there will be serious consequences to this particular case of choke, just by virtue of its persistence.

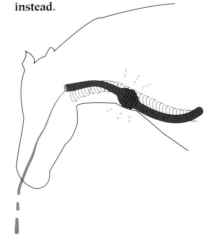

3. The longer the obstruction sits in the esophagus, the more irritated the delicate lining of the esophagus becomes. Advanced or prolonged irritation can lead to erosion and ulceration. If the damage is severe enough, the scar tissue that results when the lesions heal days later will cause a constriction in the esophagus — this will obviously leave the horse predisposed to choking again and again.

4. If a constriction occurs, future meals and drinks might cause the esophagus above the constriction to stretch out to one side, forming a sort of pelican sac, where parts of those meals can accumulate and remain until, hopefully, they manage to funnel their way through the narrowed tunnel below. Over time, this sac will become well-established and of impressive size, because it becomes the path of least resistance. The sac is called a diverticulum, because the food is *diverted* from its usual path. Some of the food retained in the sac might never drain out, becoming hardened and rock-like. Surgery is the only recourse.

5. In the worst-case scenario, the damage to the esophagus from the obstruction and/or from heavy-handed efforts to resolve it, can cause a rip. This is catastrophic, allowing the mixture of chewed food and saliva to leak out into the surrounding tissues and set up a raging infection, and making repair difficult, expensive, and often unsuccessful.

What would a vet do?

Although the diagnosis of choke is pretty obvious from a distance, the sharp veterinarian will take steps to confirm it and to rule out any other possible conditions causing similar symptoms. If the choke is located in the portion of the esophagus between jaw and chest, the vet should be able to feel it. However, half the length of the esophagus is concealed within the chest, out of reach of veterinary fingers, and the choke might be there. In this case, the vet can make the diagnosis by attempting to pass a stomach tube — if the tube encounters the obstruction, the choke is diagnosed and, as a bonus, its location is identified. Further confirmation, if necessary, can be had by passing a flexible fiberoptic scope (endoscope) that allows the examiner to actually see the obstruction.

Treatment is focused on removing the obstruction without traumatizing the delicate, easily damaged esophagus. Veterinarians that try to "ram" the obstruction with the end of the stomach tube are risking severe damage to the esophagus. The preferred treatment is to sedate the horse, then insert a stomach tube, blowing air into it to balloon the esophagus while advancing the tube until it encounters the obstruction. Small amounts of warm water are first pumped in, then aspirated back, to and fro, through the tube to soak and dissolve the obstruction and suck the dissolved pieces out. The sharp veterinarian will infuse only small amounts of water at a time — if too much is put in, the overflow can back up into the throat where it has a chance to go down the windpipe (trachea) and cause pneumonia.

If the obstruction is in the "reachable" section of the neck, gentle external massage is also done to help relax the muscles around the choke, knead the lavaging water into the obstructing material, and encourage the wad to collapse or crumble. Most chokes resolve with this treatment.

If the choke is stubborn, the vet should refrain from prolonged efforts to resolve it because of the potential for trauma to the esophagus from prolonged treatment. Instead, the horse should be muzzled to prevent eating and allowed to "rest" for

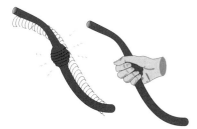

The longer a choke persists, the more the muscles of the esophagus clench around it, like a fist, making it more difficult for the obstruction to pass.

When treating a choke, it's easy to be too rough and cause more damage. Think of the esophagus as a delicate silk stocking, and the obstruction as a piece of granite. The goal is to remove the granite without snagging the stocking.

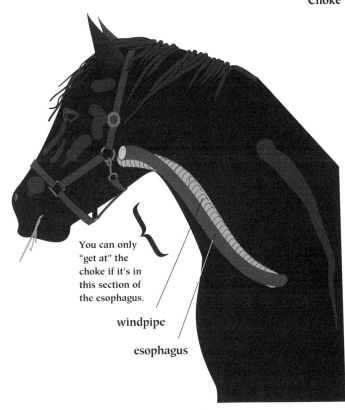

The esophagus starts just above the voicebox and passes to the left side of the neck. In most horses it stays on the left side all the way down to where the neck joins the chest. The esophagus and the windpipe (trachea) are close neighbors. Any regurgitated materials that back up out of the esophagus can easily spill down the windpipe and cause pneumonia. If the horse's head is lowered, however, and with luck, the regurgitated material will spill out onto the ground instead.

You can only "get at" the choke if it's in this section of the esophagus.

windpipe

esophagus

several hours before resuming the to-and-fro lavage treatment. If necessary, intravenous fluids and electrolytes are given during this rest period to prevent dehydration and help moisten the obstruction and the surrounding esophageal tissues from the inside.

On the second try, the vet would be wise to opt for general anesthesia to fully relax the muscles around the obstruction. Very few chokes fail to resolve this way. If, however, surgery is necessary to relieve the choke, it is historically successful only if the choke is located "up high," in the portion of the esophagus between jaw and chest. If it's any lower than that, open-chest surgery is required, and as if that weren't complicated enough, post-surgical constriction of the esophagus in this area is practically guaranteed.

After the choke has been resolved, dietary restrictions might be imposed because the muscles around the obstruction can continue to spasm, sometimes *for days* after the choke was resolved, and if the horse is put back on regular feed, rechoking is unacceptably likely. It all depends on how traumatized the tissues are from the choke and the treatment. If dietary restrictions are warranted, they can range from minor (withhold solid food for less than 24 hours) to major (feed only soft, grazed grass and sloppy mashes for 72 hours), depending on the severity of the choke and the aggressiveness of the treatment.

Antiinflammatory medications are given to sooth the inflamed tissues and reduce their reactionary spasming. However, intravenous phenylbutazone should be

Even when the choke has been resolved, the irritated esophageal muscles around the obstruction site can continue to spasm and clench for days afterwards. This makes re-choking very likely, unless the diet is adjusted during this fragile period.

avoided because it is extremely caustic and can cause rampant inflammation in the tissues of the neck if even a tiny bit leaks out of the vein (or, worse, if the person giving the injection accidentally "misses" the vein and pumps the stuff directly into the tissues). Oral phenylbutazone should also be avoided, as it can be directly irritating to the tissues of the esophagus — the last thing this horse needs. Therefore, the sharp veterinarian will choose drugs like Banamine™ or Ketofen™ which can be given intramuscularly or which, when given intravenously, are less likely to cause irritation of the tissues around the vein if leakage occurs.

The vet should also check the horse for any signs of aspiration pneumonia from inhaling regurgitated food or lavage water before or during treatment. Ultrasound and x-ray examination of the chest are valuable tools in this regard.

There's no vet. What should you do?

STEP 1.
Allow nothing by mouth.

Remove all bedding, water and food — many horses will continue to eat while choked, which will only make the choke worse and increase the risk of aspiration pneumonia.

STEP 2.
CALM...

In many cases, simply calming the horse, denying access to food, and relaxing the muscles around the obstruction will resolve the problem. Try the calming techniques described later in this chapter.

STEP 3.
Try to locate and massage the blockage.

Gently feel the esophagus (it's usually in the furrow along the left side of the neck next to the left jugular vein) and see if you can feel a lump. That lump will consist of the obstruction plus the unusually hardened, contracted muscles of the esophagus that have closed around it. If you can feel the obstruction, try to gently massage it to relax the muscles and to work the soft wad into a smaller size that can more easily pass down into the stomach. Do not try to "milk" the obstruction down toward the stomach — you may succeed only in pushing the whole thing out of reach, and you'll have lost your only direct access. Instead, gently milk it upward, in the "wrong" direction, while trying to spread it out and make it easier to pass.

STEP 4.
Hold the course.

If regurgitation continues, resist the urge to walk the horse, even though you think this might help get his mind off his discomfort. When walking, he's much more likely to become alerted to his surroundings, and he'll lift his head up to look around. This increases the risk of aspiration pneumonia. It might make *you* feel better to see the horse looking bright and alert, but what he really needs right now is to keep his head down so any regurgitating material can drain safely out his nose and onto the ground instead of going down the windpipe.

A TRAGIC CASE OF MISDIAGNOSIS

Don't be so sure about a diagnosis that you fail to make careful observations — sometimes your knowledge and experience can make you closed-minded, and your horse will suffer for it. This caveat applies just as strongly to veterinarians as it does to non-veterinary horse owners, and it is a very good reason why you should get your stricken horse to a competent equine practitioner as soon as possible. True case in point:

While their regular veterinarian was out of town, the owners of a beautiful 2-year-old Arabian filly awoke one morning to find her standing in the corner of her stall with copious volumes of "greenish slime" pouring from both nostrils. They called the only veterinarian they could find, and after one quick glance from across the fence he was *sure* of his diagnosis: Strangles — a bacterial infection of the upper respiratory tract that causes swelling of the lymph nodes under the chin, runny nose, coughing, lack of appetite, depression, and fever. A hands-on examination of the filly was not done, because the vet was worried that he might become contaminated with the highly contagious infection and spread it to other horses in the community. He advised the owners to give penicillin shots and to place a dishpan of bleach water at the doorway to the stall to disinfect their boots after medicating her, and then he left.

Three days later the regular veterinarian returned to town, and the owners asked him to check their filly, as she seemed no better. The "Strangles" was actually an advanced case of choke — the green discharge seen coming from the filly's nostrils three days earlier was regurgitated food, not "snotty nose," and a closer examination at that time would have revealed no swollen lymph nodes, no fever, no Strangles. This filly didn't need penicillin — she needed someone to remove the wad of oats that had gotten stuck in her esophagus. By this late date, however, that wad of oats had become near-concrete, and the walls of the esophagus around the obstruction had become raw and ulcerated.

To relieve the choke, which was out of reach in the lower part of the esophagus, the filly was given a general anesthetic — this caused total relaxation of the muscles that had clenched around the choke, and it permitted the veterinarian to lubricate and gently push the obstruction into the stomach where the normal digestive acids quickly broke it down. She awoke from the anesthetic and seemed fine for over a week. However, the damage to the esophagus had been extensive, and as the lesions healed and the scar tissue contracted (that's what scar tissue does at it "matures" — it shrinks), the lumen of the damaged section of esophagus became narrower and narrower. This beautiful, perfectly healthy filly developed a constriction of the esophagus, and after suffering repeated episodes of choke that became more frequent and more serious with time despite a special diet and antiinflammatory medications, and after numerous consultations with veterinary surgical specialists, she was deemed "hopeless." Out of options, the owners had her put to sleep.

While trying to lavage the obstruction, the sharp veterinarian will infuse only small amounts of warm water at a time — too much water will only contribute to the backflow and increase the chance of aspiration pneumonia.

MASSAGE: A SAFE TRANQUILIZER AND MUSCLE RELAXANT THAT REQUIRES NO PRESCRIPTION

Here's a massage technique that's custom-made for the choked horse — it can relax him and get him to lower his head. Don't be quick to pooh-pooh it: it's remarkably effective with many chokes, and it means no needles, no medicines, no money, no dangerous side-effects. Watch closely for evidence that he likes what you're doing — just like people, you'll find that some horses find a particular stroke relaxing while others find it ticklish or threatening. The EAR RUB will not be appropriate if it reminds him of earlier years when he was "eared" for restraint (some brute grabbed an ear and twisted it, using this for restraint in lieu of a regular twitch) — if that's the case with your horse, just stick with the SCALP LIFT and stay away from the ears.

How do you know if you're having the right effect? If he lowers his head, takes a deep breath and sighs heavily, gets a sleepy, dreamy look in his eye, lets his lips droop, or starts slowly chewing, you're on the right track.

How do you know if he's not relaxing? If he raises his head to the "alert" or "buzz off" position, moves away from you, looks at you sideways (maybe even showing a little eye white), swishes his tail, or generally tenses up. It might be that you're just not being gentle enough. Try backing off and starting over with a lighter touch, or, if you think he's just not keen about having any activity around his head, just switch to rubbing or currying him in the brisket. Remember, in addition to calming him, you also want his head lowered. Although most horses love having their back and withers scratched, some horses tend to raise their heads in appreciation — not the effect you're going for. You can try it in your horse, but quit if he lifts his head.

STEP 5.
Apply hot packs.

Apply warm, moist compresses to the obstruction for ten minutes at a time to help sooth and relax the contracted muscles. A washcloth soaked in warm water and squeezed out is adequate, or a chemical hot pack will do.

A chemical hot pack held over the blockage can help relax the spasming muscles.

STEP 6.
Think you've got it? Check it out.

If at any point you think the obstruction might be relieved, test your theory by wiping the horse's muzzle clean with a soft cloth and offering water: he is likely to be thirsty and will probably give it a try, and you can watch his nostrils closely for any water spilling back out. If you see water coming out, stop him and remove the water source until further evidence that he's in the clear.

1. Stand on his left side and brush, curry, or work your fingers into the coat along the side of the neck. Work your way down to the brisket (in the front between the front legs) and let him appreciate your touch in this area where he can never scratch himself. Do this for as long as he enjoys it, particularly if he lowers his head. (Caution: some stallions find this to be sexually provocative. If in doubt, skip it.)

2. Place your right hand about 6 inches forward of the withers by the crest of the mane. Burrow your fingers affectionately into the hair coat and spend a minute working the surface tissues with your fingertips as though gently but firmly trying to work up a lather while shampooing.

3. Gradually work up the crest of the neck until you're at the poll behind the right ear — take at least a minute to make the journey.

4. Stay at the poll for a minute or two and gently but assertively work the thick skin there, pushing it around in half-dollar-sized circles, but steering clear of the ears.

5. Gently tug tufts of mane hair behind the ears: lift straight up, pulling the scalp slightly off the skull, then letting it back down. Most horses LOVE this, and the head will come down even more.

6. Now work your hand to the base of the ear, gently pushing the thick cartilage where the ear joins the head slightly back and forth between thumb and fingers. Do this for two minutes. Keep your fingers out of the inside of the ear unless he's accustomed to it. The muscles that normally hold the ear erect will relax and soften.

7. Now fold the edges of the ear together and "milk" upward in a single, slow, relaxed motion, as though pushing soft toothpaste out of a tube, releasing your grip just before you get to the tip of the ear. Do this for a minute. Be gentle. Work the ear in its current position, rather than pulling it up or out to the side. If he seems to object, go back to step 6 to regain his confidence, then try step 7 again. Still no good? That's okay — just stick with steps 4 through 6.

The brisket rub

The poll mover

The scalp lift

The ear rub

If you do the water test and no water regurgitation occurs at the nostrils, congratulations—you may be out of the woods. However, you're not off the hook. For at least the next 24-72 hours (depending on how he does during that period), his diet should be altered to soothe his irritated esophagus and minimize the chances of a repeat episode. Feed soft grazed grass (15-minute grazing sessions), sloppy mashes, or soaked hay cubes (soaked long enough to make a sloppy gruel but not long enough that the

STEP 7.

Adjust the diet for the healing period.

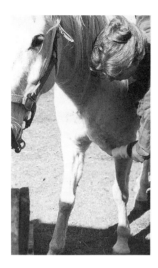 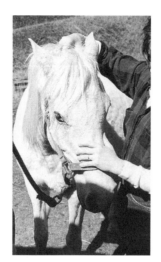 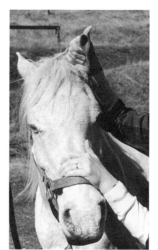 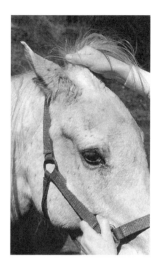

Left to right:
the brisket rub, the poll mover,
the ear rub, and the hair pull

In treating the choked horse, it's essential to get him to relax so that the muscles of his neck will soften and so he'll lower his head to allow any regurgitated materials to drain out, rather than spill into his windpipe. For some horses, a gentle currying in the brisket area is just the ticket. Others appreciate a soothing massage of the external ear, folding it in half lengthwise and running the hand upward, from base to tip, in a repetitive, firm stroke. For those that hate having their ears "messed with," an especially popular method is the scalp lift: work your fingers into the strands of hair at the forelock and just behind the ears, then, by curling the fingers and gripping the hair at its base, gently lift the skin of the scalp slightly from the skull, then release. Humans appreciate this as well — try it!

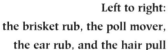

SPECIAL NOTE 10.1

You might be tempted to give the choked horse a sedative to relax him, release his muscular grip on the obstruction, and get him to lower his head. Don't do it. Sedatives can interfere with the normal swallowing reflex and predispose the horse to aspiration pneumonia. Besides, if you end up having to take him to a vet for his choke, the last thing you want is a "drugged," staggering horse in a moving horse trailer.

whole mess spoils), and offer water separately. Keep a close eye on his nostrils for evidence of regurgitation and also watch the "whole horse" for evidence of the original signs of choke. If it appears that he can handle his usual daily amount of food, divide it into ten or more multiple small meals so he never gets the chance to get ravenously hungry (which would encourage bolting) and so each snack has a good chance to be well chewed, savored, and successfully swallowed. The smaller meal also has the advantage of causing only brief scratching of the already irritated esophagus, giving its reactionary spasms time to relax and quiet down before the next little meal. Wait at least twelve hours before offering any hay, and make the first hay offerings very small and very high-quality: just enough leafy, fine-stemmed hay to loosely fill a standard shoebox. If that small amount is well received and no regurgitation or discomfort is seen (be sure to LOOK), it can be repeated every one to two hours until 24-72 hours have passed *and* no mishaps have occurred. Depending on what you decide was the cause of this choke, you might also want to consider a total overhaul of your horse's management and diet to prevent future episodes.

If after a full hour of gentle massage, warm moist compresses, and "starvation," your horse is still choked, the odds that this is a serious choke with dangerous consequences are unacceptably high, and he'll be better off in the trailer (NO HAY) headed for the nearest competent equine veterinarian, no matter *how* far away that might be.

STEP 8.
No luck? Hit the road.

Whether you've succeeded in resolving the choke or not, give an intramuscular injection of Banamine™ (see *Special Note 10.2* for dose) to ward off excessive inflammation of the irritated esophagus. By abbreviating the inflammation, you'll cut short the period of muscle spasming, and you'll decrease the chance that the horse will re-choke while he's in the recovery phase.

STEP 9.
Give an antiinflammatory.

Should you seek veterinary assistance?

Yes, because even if you resolved the choke, you have no way of knowing whether your horse aspirated any regurgitated material into his lungs.

SPECIAL NOTE 10.2

DOSAGE RECOMMENDATION FOR BANAMINE™ IN CHOKE

800 lb horse	3cc
900 lb horse	3½ cc
1000 lb horse	4 cc
1100 lb horse	4 cc
1200 lb horse	4½ cc
1300 lb horse	4½ cc
1400 lb horse	5 cc

To be given intramuscularly, once only.

CHAPTER 11

The Troubled Eye

Your horse's eye is watering, red, squinted nearly closed. Perhaps even his eyelids are swollen. As you set the hay net down and try to decide what to do, he walks toward the open stall door where you're standing, shoves his head through the opening, and starts rhythmically raking the swollen tissues of his face across the edge of the doorway. Horrified, you shout at him to stop, which he does, but only temporarily. A steady stream of clear tears is running from between his clenched eyelids.

Serious eye ailments, whether from injury or disease process, are nothing to play with — whatever your current situation is, the recommendations that follow are meant only as stop-gap measures to get the crisis under control until you can get the horse into the hands of the nearest competent equine veterinarian.

What's causing the problem?

The most common emergency eye problems include:

Any eye incident can set the stage for recurrent uveitis, also known as moon blindness, a nagging, painful condition that threatens blindness every time it shows up.

Trouble in the eye itself

- Foreign material on the eye (dust, grit, weed seeds, chaff, etc)
- Non-penetrating eye wound (a scratch)
- Penetrating eye wound (a poke)
- Infection of the eyeball's outer "shell" (a corneal ulcer)
- Blunt trauma to the eyeball (a whollop)
- Uveitis and recurrent uveitis (Moon Blindness)

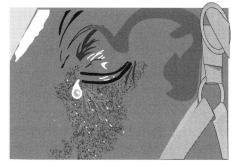

- Foreign material in the pockets around the eye (dust, grit, weed seeds, chaff, etc.)
- Injury to the tissues around the eye
- Blunt trauma to the tissues around the eye (a whollop)

What you see

Most of the major emergency eye conditions look alike from the outside: the inflamed eye is painful and sensitive to the light, the eyelids are blinking or clamped shut, clear tears are spilling down the horse's face, there might also be some thicker, whitish discharge, the normally clear cornea might look fogged, and the horse may be rubbing the eye.

What's going on inside, and why is this dangerous?

The most common eye problem in the horse is a scratch, poke, or whollop to the clear, outer globe called the cornea, thanks to the anatomy of the head that makes the horse's large, prominent, sticking-out-to-the-sides eyeballs especially vulnerable to injury. Fresh, noninfected, superficial corneal injuries are usually accompanied by only mild to moderate squinting and watering — the pain resolves quickly with prompt, appropriate treatment (and often without it), and the injury can heal in as quickly as a day or two.

But if the cornea becomes infected, a quick, uncomplicated recovery is not in the cards. If the infection were elsewhere in the body, high-tech antibodies would quickly arrive at the site of the infection via the bloodstream. But the cornea has no blood supply — that's why it's clear. It's nourished by seepage of nutrients through its onion-like layers from the liquids that bathe it inside the eyeball. This gives invading bacteria an advantage, a chance to get established before the eye figures out a way to get a sophisticated immune response to the battlefield — there are some crude infection-fighters inside the eyeball, but the "big guns" from the bloodstream are needed for more serious infections, and without help, they just might not get there in time.

To make matters worse, some bacteria (such as *Pseudomonas* species) have the ability to secrete chemicals that can literally melt away the structure of the cornea — unchecked, they can destroy the eyeball in a matter of a day or two. Scrambling to protect itself, the eyeball will build a network of blood vessels on the cornea to help fight the infection, sacrificing the clear-glass structure of the cornea in order to save the eye. But this hasty effort takes days, it's sloppy and haphazard, and even if the infection is defeated, the eye is likely to be permanently marred with ugly, vision-impairing patches of opaque scar tissue.

If the corneal injury is deep, contaminated, or accompanied by additional trauma to the eye, the external signs of discomfort can be quite profound because of a reaction that will occur inside the eye: the muscle that controls the size of the pupil

Thanks to a serious infection within its onion-like layers, this mare's cornea is now thickly and permanently scarred, and even though the rest of the eye is fine, she's unable to see through all the scar tissue.

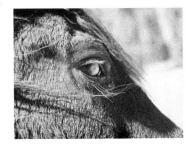

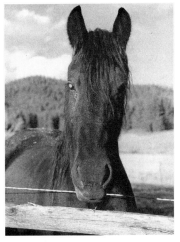

Even when the problem is as innocent as dust in the eye, persistent eye pain is so universally unbearable that most horses will rub. Severe damage is as close as the nearest rough-hewn post, the nearest protruding nail, the nearest creosote-treated board... just waiting to make the acquaintance of a delicate eyeball.

will spasm with pain, the pupil will become significantly smaller, and a sort of inflammatory bonfire will start inside the eye. This is called *uveitis*.

Uveitis is extremely painful, like a migraine headache inside the eyeball, and even after the underlying problem has been solved, the excruciating spasm of that muscle can become self-perpetuating. How or why this happens is not yet understood, but a one-time bout with an eye problem of any sort can turn into a chronic condition called recurrent uveitis or *Moon Blindness*, where the uveitis returns with no warning and for no apparent reason. Each recurrence can do sufficient damage to the internal structures of the eye to blind the horse permanently, unless recognized quickly and aggressively treated.

Meanwhile, any eye tissues that are within reach of contaminating bacteria can be invaded, setting the stage for more inflammation as the immune system inside the eyeball tries to fight off the invasion while summoning reinforcements from the general bloodstream.

If any debris from the ensuing fracas manages to clog up the eyeball's plumbing system, the eyeball itself will begin to enlarge from an overall increase in pressure with nowhere to drain off the excess. This is called glaucoma, and, like uveitis, it threatens permanent damage, possibly blindness.

Furthermore, if the inflammation inside the eyeball is severe, adhesions can form between inner components such as the lens and the iris (the colored part of the eye). If this happens, the pupil will be stuck to the lens, unable to widen or constrict in response to light.

Even when the underlying cause is something as innocent as dust in the eye, persistent eye pain is so unbearable that the horse is likely to rub, and he's not likely to do it very carefully or delicately, nor is he going to select a clean, safe object to rub against — he'll use a door jamb, a hay rack, a splintery rough-hewn post, maybe even his own filthy hoof. As a result, an eye that started out with a simple and easily resolved problem can end up badly traumatized.

THE GOAL

So the goal in treating any eye problem is:

- to prevent or reverse uveitis,
- to prevent or reverse infection,
- to prevent self-trauma by eliminating discomfort and foiling the horse's attempts to rub, and
- to encourage rapid healing with a minimum of scar tissue.

What would the vet do?

In the ideal situation, the underlying cause of the eye problem is identified and corrected, the corruption of the eye is halted, the damaged tissues are repaired, and with sophisticated medications and equipment, the eye is kept comfortable and

The clear, glass-like cornea should have no fogginess, white spots or blood vessels.

Shine a flashlight into a horse's eye and you should see 3 reflections: from the cornea, the front of the lens, and the back of the lens.

The lumpy corpus nigrum is an extra "awning" to shade the retina from the sun.

The pupil is a horizontal oval in the horse.

The sclera, or "white of the eye," is usually hidden unless you tilt the horse's head to have a look.

The "third eyelid," or nictitating membrane usually stays open, tucked in the inside corner of the eye. If it's pulled over the eye in the awake horse, there's a problem.

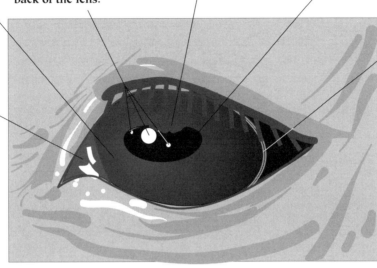

otherwise protected against self-trauma until healing is complete.

However, the horse's defensive reflexes aren't about to allow anybody, no matter who he is and what his credentials might be, to open those eyelids, touch those tender tissues, and have a look while shining bright lights inside. Furthermore, some of the procedures the vet might need to do might require the use of sharp instruments, maybe even needles, around the eye, and if the horse doesn't hold absolutely still (and who would, under the circumstances), the possibility for more serious damage is very real.

So the veterinarian starts the eye exam by disabling the horse's defense mechanisms, using one or more of several "weapons": sedation, general anesthesia, topical numbing agents to deaden the surface of the eye, nerve blocks to deaden the tissues in and around the eye, and nerve blocks to disable the powerful "blink" reflexes and keep the eyeball from moving around.

Once that's accomplished, the eye and surrounding tissues are carefully cleaned, usually by repeated flushing with eye-safe solutions, and finally the real eye exam can get under way, using special magnifying lenses, surgical-quality lighting, dyes, and instruments designed to pull the eyelids away from the eye so the examiner can get a look into the dark pockets and corners where pokers and grit and other foreign matter can hide. If infection is suspected, samples might be taken for laboratory culture and analysis. Treatment should be carefully tailored according to what the examination reveals, and because the horse is in a controlled environment,

One of the veterinarian's biggest advantages in dealing with traumatized eyes is the nerve block. With a swift, skillfully placed injection, he/she can deaden the pain, immobilize the eye, and stop that infernal eyelid from clamping down. These defense mechanisms are your biggest problem when you're out in the middle of nowhere and your horse has an eye problem — he won't even let you look, let alone touch.

Many equine eyes are decimated by the do-it-yourself remedies commonly recommended by well-meaning but misinformed horsemen.

DON'T FORCE IT!
If the injury is severe, the added pressure of a tightly clenched eyelid trying to fight your efforts to pry it open can actually rupture the eyeball.

The good news

Don't be surprised if, in spite of signs of severe eye pain, you see no evidence of any external eye trauma. Your horse could be suffering from an attack of uveitis — an invisible "bonfire" inside his eye.

keeping his eye medicated and keeping him from traumatizing his tender orbs is a relatively straightforward matter of choosing one of several devices to protect him from himself.

There's no vet. What should you do?

But here you are, away from home, no vet available, and the environment is anything but controlled. A thorough examination of a painful eye is probably not going to be possible, owing to those powerful defense mechanisms the horse is going to use to keep you away from the source of his pain, and the fact that you don't have all the tools or any of the training the veterinarian has to overcome those defenses.

Furthermore, should you persist in your efforts to have a look by force, you run the risk of doing a great deal more damage. An eye that has been "wholloped," for example, or one that is suffering from a dangerous corneal infection, might be so weakened that the added pressure of a tightly clenched eyelid, trying to fight your efforts to force it open, might actually cause the eyeball to rupture.

Your goals, then, will be to make the eye more comfortable, to relieve some of the secondary inflammation and swelling, to prevent self-induced trauma from blinking and rubbing, and, if it's not a simple case that resolves right away, to transfer the case to the vet as soon as possible.

Believe it or not, despite all this scary talk about blindness and ruptured eyeballs, there's good news for your squinting, teary-eyed horse:

1. The vast majority of mild to moderate squinty, watery eye conditions will resolve almost immediately if you follow the instructions given in this chapter.

2. More severe cases are quickly recognizable because of their lack of response. In other words, you won't have to guess how "bad" it is — you'll know within a few hours whether this is a complicated case that requires special veterinary attention. This is good. It means that there's little chance of prolonged delays in recognizing the gravity of the situation.

More importantly, even though you weren't able to "cure" the problem yourself, your treatments will have relieved some of the inflammation and swelling, making it easier for the veterinarian to see what's going on inside, and making the horse more comfortable and less likely to further traumatize the eye by rubbing.

Equally important: if you follow the instructions in this chapter, you will have avoided any treatments that might have made the situation worse — many equine eyes are decimated by the do-it-yourself remedies commonly recommended by well-meaning but misinformed horsemen.

The Three Plans of Attack

Your horse's eye discomfort is mild to moderate if he holds the eye at least 50% open when not being "messed with," and if the tissues around the eye show no signs of swelling or external trauma from rubbing. If your horse's case fits this category, do the following:

Without touching the eye, try to get a look by tricking the horse into opening the eye completely (make a distracting noise, for example, or shake an interesting looking object such as a tissue or plastic bag, or rustle some oats in a bucket). By holding his head still and moving an interesting object from one end of his field of vision to the other, you can "trick" him into exposing his entire eyeball, including the top, bottom, inside and outside margins. Raise his head by pushing his chin up, and examine the upper margin of the eyeball exposed when he rolls his eye downward.

Now, since his discomfort is on the lower end of the scale, you can attempt to get a closer look. To examine his left eye, stand on his left side and pull his nose toward you by pulling on the halter with your right hand, and hold it steady by laying your left elbow over the top of his muzzle . Gently but firmly place your left hand over his eye, your index finger on his upper lid and your thumb on his lower lid, and gently press into the eyeball so the lids open. Take a look inside:

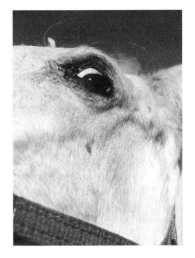

By pushing the chin up, you can get a "free" look at the upper margins of the eye.

PLAN 1: For mild to moderate eye discomfort with no swelling of the tissues around the eye

If you see foreign material (such as weed seeds or chaff) on the eye, you'll need to flush it out with an eyewash solution. The horse is likely to resent this. Make your job easier by warming the eyewash solution to a comfortable, room-temperature level — he's sure to fight you if the rinse is cold. And, of course, don't get it too warm. Warm

STEP 1a.

SPECIAL NOTE 11.1

If you need to numb the eye in order to flush out foreign material, you can apply a drop or two of a topical anesthetic, made just for eyes — this is a prescription item, to be procured from your veterinarian only for emergencies. There are two hazards of topical eye anesthetics:

1. They can retard the healing process and, therefore, should only be used once, so you can examine the eye — they're not meant to be used over and over, to relieve the pain.

2. Bacteria and fungi love these solutions. Therefore, get only a tiny bottle, use it one time only, and throw the rest away. After it's been opened, what remains in the bottle is almost certain to be contaminated, and since you'll only be using it on eyes that have been traumatized, you surely don't want to risk causing an infection.

---

it by dunking the sealed bottle in a bowl of lukewarm water, and check the temperature before using it on your horse's eye. If you think it might be too warm, it probably is.

If the horse just won't tolerate it because of his pain, you can apply a drop or two of proparacaine solution to numb the eye, giving it a minute or two to take effect (see *Special Note 11.1*). Then flood the eye with the eye wash solution until the foreign material is washed out.

When you're sure the eye is clean, squeeze a line of triple antibiotic ophthalmic ointment right across the eyeball, being careful to "plant" your hands against his face so you won't poke the eye with the tip of the tube if he moves (see *Special Note 11.4*).

STEP 1b. **If you see nothing to explain the eye's discomfort,** squeeze a line of triple antibiotic ophthalmic ointment directly across the eyeball, and, just beneath that line, squeeze a line of atropine ophthalmic ointment.

STEP 2. Confine the horse in a cool, dark place away from direct sunlight, dust, and wind for an hour. Place hay on the floor, rather than in a hay rack or net, so chaff and dust won't fall into his eyes.

STEP 3. When the hour has passed, *and without touching the eye*, check for continued discomfort. You're looking for

- watering,
- squinting,
- redness,
- rubbing, and/or
- the development of any swelling around the eye.

If any of these signs is present, the problem is more severe than you thought, and you should head for the nearest veterinary facility and/or follow the instructions below.

PLAN 2: For moderate to severe eye discomfort with or without swelling of the tissues around the eye

Your horse's eye discomfort is moderate to severe if he holds the eye clamped shut, even when not being "messed with," and/or if the tissues around the eye are swollen, possibly even traumatized from rubbing. If your horse's case fits this category, do the following:

Calm the horse by being calm yourself. Move him to a cool, quiet, darkened area away from direct sunlight, wind, dust, and protruding objects such as protruding branches. If you've put him into a stall with hay rack or net, move all hay to the floor where dust and chaff won't fall into his eyes.

SPECIAL NOTE 11.2

"BUTE" DOSE FOR EYE PAIN

800 lb horse:	1 gram
900 lb horse:	1 gram
1,000 lb horse:	1½ grams
1,100 lb horse:	1½ grams
1,200 lb horse:	1½ grams
1,300 lb horse:	2 grams
1,400 lb horse:	2 grams

To be given orally, once only.

If at all possible, do not leave him unattended until you've finished with your ministrations — at this stage, you can't trust him to not worsen the situation by rubbing.

STEP 1.

a. If the horse is extremely resentful of any efforts to look at the area, and/or if the tissues around the eye are so swollen that you couldn't open the eye even if he'd let you, treat the pain and inflammation "from a distance" and leave the eye alone: give an intramuscular injection of Banamine™ (see *Special Note 11.3*).

b. If the pain is severe: also give bute paste or gel orally (see *Special Note 11.2*).

STEP 2.

If the swelling around the eye is severe, do not try to force the swollen lids open. Instead, gently apply a cold pack directly over the swollen area and hold it there for five minutes. The horse might resist at first, but if you're gentle and gradual and persistent with your approach, he'll allow it and soon realize that it feels good.

STEP 3.

Now you're going to apply an eye patch. But first, if he'll allow it (which he might, since the antiinflammatories and ice pack have had a few minutes to work their magic), apply a line of atropine ophthalmic ointment and a line of triple antibiotic ophthalmic ointment between the edges of the swollen lids directly onto the eyeball before applying the patch — the use of a twitch might be helpful in getting the eye medicated.

If there's just no way of getting the ointments onto the eye, they can be applied to the rims of the closed eyelids or incorporated into the patch as described below — just slather a mound of both kinds of ophthalmic ointment onto a clean 4 x 4 gauze sponge and place it over the closed eye so that the bulk of the ointment contacts the eye where the lids meet. The warmth of the tissues will melt the ointment into the opening and ooze over the eyeball, protecting it from dryness and performing the essential tasks of the medications. Be sure to give *both* ointments — the atropine, and the antibiotic. Each has an essential role.

Patch the eye (see illustration later in this chapter). This will keep the lid closed, thereby eliminating the irritation from constant blinking or squinting — the eyelid can act as sandpaper, particularly if it has foreign material embedded in it. Furthermore, the closed eyelid forms an ideal natural bandage to keep the traumatized eyeball covered, warm, moist, and protected against further trauma. And if the injury is so severe that the eyeball is in danger of rupturing, the closed eyelid will help to support the eyeball.

STEP 4.

Now that the first-string treatments have been done and the eye has been protected by the bandage, the horse can be safely transported to the nearest competent equine veterinarian. Upon arrival, odds are that what the veterinarian finds under the bandage will look a lot prettier than what you saw initially, thanks to your efforts at halting and reversing the swelling, pain, redness, uveitis, contamination and infection.

SPECIAL NOTE 11.3

BANAMINE™ DOSE FOR EYE PAIN

800 lb horse:	3 cc
900 lb horse:	3 cc
1,000 lb horse:	3½ cc
1,100 lb horse:	4 cc
1,200 lb horse:	4 cc
1,300 lb horse:	4½ cc
1,400 lb horse:	5 cc

To be given intramuscularly, once only.

By planting your hands against his face, you can be sure that if the horse moves his head, your hand and the tip of the ointment tube will move right along with it, thereby preventing an accidental poke. Whenever possible, "draw a line" of ointment right across the eyeball. If he resists, try depositing it in the "pouch" behind the lower eyelid, although he's just as likely to resist that too, if he won't stand for the preferred method. If all attempts at direct medication fail, mound a glob of the ointment(s) on a stack of clean gauze sponges and press it right against the closed eye where the upper and lower lids meet, then secure the stack with a bandage.

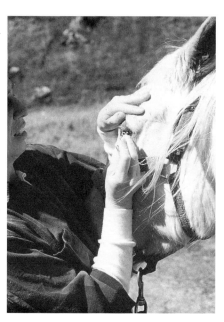

SPECIAL NOTE 11.5

If you have reason to believe that the facial bones around the eye may have been fractured (for example, if the horse collided with a solid object, such as a tree, or a wall, or another horse), see *Chapter 9*. If the trauma to his head was severe enough to break bones, it was also severe enough to risk brain injury.

If there's an unavoidable delay in getting to the veterinary facility, let the ice and the antiinflammatory medications do their work for an hour, then remove the bandage and have a look before remedicating and replacing the bandage.

After removing the head wrap, do not touch the face or the eye or otherwise arouse the horse's resentment (he'll react by clamping the lid closed), and do not expose the eye to sunlight or wind (ditto).

Give him a minute to readjust to the light, then have a hands-off look: the swelling should be reduced, and you should be able to judge his pain by assessing how widely he'll open the eye — generally, the better it feels, the wider he'll voluntarily open it.

Also check to see if it is still watering: look for drops of clear watery discharge spilling over the rims of his lower lids onto his face — this indicates that although you may have improved the situation, there's still an underlying problem going on, and you'd better renew your efforts to get him to the nearest competent equine veterinarian pronto.

Remedicate the eye for the trip: draw fresh lines of triple antibiotic ointment and atropine ointment directly across the cornea if he'll allow it, load up a fresh 4 x 4 gauze sponge with fresh mounds of triple antibiotic and atropine ophthalmic ointments, and replace, along with the cold pack and the head wrap.

The stockinette (or a leg from a men's large longjohns) makes a very good "bandage" to hold the stack of medicated gauze against a troubled eye. Just slip the stack into place after putting the stockinette on (cut holes for the "good" eye and the ears as you unroll it across his face). The patched eye will benefit from nature's best eye bandage: the closed eyelid — it's warm, moist, and completely protects the eye against sunlight, wind and dust, and when patched, the eyelid won't squint or blink and further irritate the eye. A few strategic figure-eights with a stretchy, elastic-backed bandage material (Expandover is especially good for this purpose), followed by the halter over the whole thing, will nicely secure the patch and discourage rubbing.

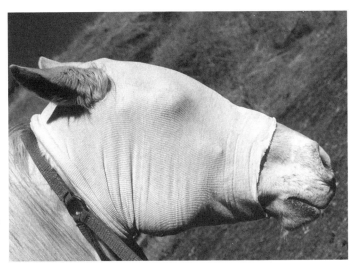

PLAN 3: For horses with a known history of recurrent uveitis (AKA "moon blindness")

A horse that has previously been diagnosed with moon blindness is prone to recurrent episodes at any time, with no warning and no apparent reason for the attacks. Each attack has the potential to cause permanent blindness, and aggressive treatment might be required. Therefore, you should not attempt to deal with it alone unless you truly have no choice.

By the same token, you should not fail to institute immediate treatment before taking steps to locate a competent and willing equine veterinarian to help your horse — time is of the essence in treating uveitis, and a delay in starting treatment just because you're timid about doing any treatments yourself can mean the difference between vision and blindness for your horse's future.

Therefore, you should see the treatment for moon blindness as a team effort: you're responsible for early detection, first-string treatment, and for getting the horse to a veterinarian as soon as possible; the vet is responsible for continuing the care you started, initiating veterinarian-only treatments (which can include the use of steroid medications and the injection of medications directly into the delicate tissues around the eyeball) and laboratory diagnostic efforts to hopefully identify and eliminate the underlying cause.

WARNING:
Do not use any eye medications that contain steroids unless specifically prescribed by a veterinarian for this specific horse and this specific problem. Why? Because steroid medications on an eye with certain types of corneal injury can encourage the damaged cornea to "melt away," resulting in permanent damage with scarring or rupture. Check the label for the words cortisol, cortisone, hydrocortisol, hydrocortisone, prednisone, prednisolone, triamcinolone, etc.

How can you tell if the pupil is constricted?

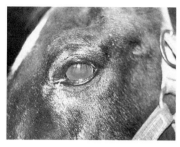

This is a constricted pupil in a horse suffering from recurrent uveitis. Atropine ophthalmic ointment has been applied to temporarily "paralyze" the spasming muscle inside the eye that is causing the pupil to close, but it hasn't been successful yet. Compared to an unaffected horse's eye in the same lighting conditions, the pupil in this eye is small.

The same horse, 24 hours later: the atropine has finally overcome the spasming muscle, and the pupil is now opened up wider than is normal. In treating uveitis, this is a good result, and the horse's eye is now much more comfortable. Note that instead of the normal shape of the pupil (a horizontal oval), the dilated pupil is large and round.

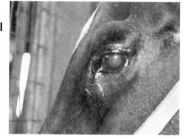

EARLY DETECTION OF UVEITIS

If uveitis has been diagnosed before in your horse, always be on the lookout for any of the following signs in one or both eyes:

- "bloodshot eyes": the whites of the eyes and the tissues around the eyeballs are "veiny" and red
- squinting
- sensitivity to light
- watery eye
- foggy cornea
- constricted pupil (see above)
- sudden blindness

First-string treatment

1. If he's outside, bring him into a stall to protect him against direct sunlight, wind, and dust. If this is not possible, apply a fine-gauge cloth screen-type fly bonnet.

2. Give Banamine™ injection intramuscularly (see *Special Note 11.3*)

3. Give "bute" gel or paste orally (see *Special Note 11.2*)

4. Draw a line of atropine ophthalmic ointment directly across the cornea

5. Draw a line of triple antibiotic ophthalmic ointment directly across the cornea

6. Locate the nearest competent equine veterinarian and get the horse hospitalized as soon as possible.

SPECIAL NOTE 11.6

Some texts recommend applying DMSO products to the lids of a traumatized eye. DO NOT DO THIS. Granted, DMSO is an excellent topical antiinflammatory, but many horses have local skin reactions to it — they behave as though it burns or stings — and in some cases they'll act almost frenzied in their attempts to scratch or rub it off. This is the last thing you need on your horse's already traumatized eye.

Tying-Up Syndrome

A problem of endurance horses, polo ponies, three-day-eventers, and other high-intensity athletes

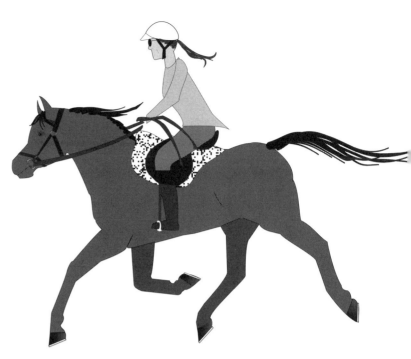

I t might have been subtle at first — a reluctance, a hesitation, a sluggishness. Now it's obvious that something's wrong: your horse's muscles are stiffening up.

Myositis.

Your riding partner says to walk your horse until he loosens up. Your friend, who works pit crew for you during races, says he heard that walking is the worst thing you can do. There's no veterinarian available. What should you do?

It's known by several names: myositis, tying-up syndrome, rhabdomyolysis, Monday morning disease, azoturia — they all translate to a dangerous muscle disorder that is most often, if not exclusively, a problem of the working, performance horse. It's an occupational hazard for equine athletes.

Many cases of muscle disorder occur at the site of a competition, where a competent equine veterinarian is already on the grounds. Unfortunately, though, just as many cases occur during training, or on the way to an event, or on the way back from an event, where the problem is just as dangerous and just as likely to blow up with improper treatment. Certain individual horses, particularly those with a high-strung, anxious tendency to get excited when anticipating an event, can get hit with a major muscle disorder just about any time, anywhere, including (especially) when there's no vet available for 100 miles.

This chapter is for situations like these, and for horse people who simply want to understand why the vet does what he/she does when the problem occurs at an event. If you're on your own, use the information in this chapter to exercise damage control, to stop the cascade of destructive events occurring in your horse's muscles, and to keep his condition stable or, preferably, improve it, while you're trying to locate a veterinarian who can take over for you as soon as possible.

What you see

The most common finding is a stiff, stilted gait that is obviously not due to a single-leg lameness — the whole horse is stiff.

The mild case: The signs will be subtle in a mildly affected horse — he might show only a poor performance or a lack of impulsion rather than any obvious soreness, and it's only after a closer look that you recognize the problem: he doesn't really want to move, and his muscles feel tense and hard.

The moderate case: The moderately affected horse will, in addition to showing more obvious muscle tenderness and stiffness, have rapid, labored breathing. Also, he may flinch when you press on the major muscles of the croup, loins, thighs, and along the spine.

The severe case: In severe cases, the cramping, spasming muscle activity is actually visible from the outside, creating a confusing picture of profuse sweating, pain and a look of anxiety — in fact, it's often mistaken for colic. What sets it apart from colic, however, is that the major muscles feel tense and hard to your fingers, the horse is extremely resentful of finger pressure on those major muscles, and his urine, should you be lucky enough to see it, is becoming increasingly dark colored, as though it has been laced with weak coffee. The heart and respiratory rates are elevated, the rectal temperature is above normal, and a flood of endotoxins is entering the bloodstream from dying muscle fibers.

What's causing his muscles to stiffen?

Well, that depends. There are really only two main categories of serious muscle disorder:

- **Type A:** The symptoms in this kind of muscle disorder occur suddenly, *early* in a workout, long before the horse has significantly exerted himself. This is often referred to as "Monday morning syndrome," and what's happening on the inside is that the fibers in the stricken muscles are actually breaking apart. This type of myositis is often seen in polo ponies, three-day eventers, and sprinters.

- **Type B:** The symptoms in this kind of muscle disorder occur more gradually, later in a workout, *after* the horse has significantly exerted himself. In some cases, the signs don't even show up until the competitive event is over. This type of myositis is typical of the endurance horse and the harness racer.

It's important that you decide which of these categories your horse's condition fits into, because you'll handle them differently. How to differentiate them will be

Severe cases of myositis are often mistaken for colic — they show the same profuse sweating, severe unfocused pain, and anxiety.

There are two types of myositis: Type A and Type B. It's important that you figure out which type your horse has, because they're handled differently.

explained later in this section.

Why is this condition dangerous?

There's much more to it than just stiff, sore muscles—this is a bodywide disorder that is expressing itself in other places in the body as well as the muscles, and if it's not handled correctly the horse's career in competition is over. In severe cases, management of myositis can arrest the damage, or, if handled improperly, it can spread it and threaten the horse's performance future, maybe even threaten his life.

Type A Myositis

In the case of Type A myositis, where the muscle fibers are degenerating, the broken-down muscle cells create a "toxic waste dump" inside the horse's body, with the major offending toxins being myoglobin and an endotoxin known as LPS (lipopolysaccharides).

The *LPS toxins* leak into the system during the stress of major exertion, and they cause changes in the circulation that seem to be self-defeating: the heart becomes less efficient at pumping blood, the breathing becomes labored, and the blood vessels feeding the major muscles become constricted, thereby depriving the muscles of the very blood they need to do their job. If significantly deprived in this manner, the muscles will begin to die, fiber by fiber. Horses that are younger and have had less experience with the rigors of high-stress exertion seem more vulnerable to the effects of these toxins, and a recent study gives us a hint at why that might be: With each training experience, the body's immune system becomes "introduced" to small amounts of the LPS toxin leaking from damaged muscles, and it responds to that introduction by building antibodies to cancel out the toxin's effects. Veteran racehorses have high levels of the anti-toxin antibodies circulating in their bloodstream, making them better able to deactivate higher doses of the toxin. Newcomers to the competitive scene, however, are virtually unprotected, and they are much more likely to suffer the consequences if they're asked to over-exert during this "competition-naïve" stage of their lives. Type A myositis is one of those consequences.

Myoglobin is a major by-product of muscle breakdown, and the only way the body can eliminate myoglobin from the body is through the urine. That's why the urine of a myositis-stricken horse has a coffee-colored discoloration: it contains myoglobin, which is reddish-brown. Trouble is, the particles of myoglobin are really too large to be handled properly by the delicate filtration system of the kidneys, and when the kidneys are suddenly barraged with massive loads of the stuff, their filters get clogged up. So the horse with Type A myositis, in addition to suffering massive muscle loss (which threatens his competitive future) is also at risk of suffering kidney shutdown (which threatens his life).

This is a bodywide disorder — it's not just in the muscles — and if it's not handled correctly, your horse's career could be over.

Type B Myositis

In Type B myositis, the muscle disorder is part of a broader spectrum of problems, including dehydration, electrolyte imbalance, depletion of muscle energy stores, and, in some cases, accumulation of lactic acid in the muscles — all factors that are much more likely to occur in horses that are inadequately conditioned prior to an event, and/or horses that are pushed too hard and not allowed to slow the pace when they show the subtle, early signs of exhaustion. The body reacts to the deficiency of fluids and specific electrolytes by shutting down the blood vessels to the major muscles, and if those blood vessels are permitted to stay closed, the muscles begin to suffocate, spasm, and die.

What would the vet do?

The sharp veterinarian would start by shouting, "Freeze!" Further movement of horses with Type A muscle problems will only increase their pain and magnify their muscle damage. Slow, in-hand walking is sometimes advocated for horses with Type B muscle problems, but before the vet can make a recommendation in this regard, he/she will need a chance to examine the horse and decide which type of problem he has.

TYPE A

If the diagnosis is Type A, the vet would confirm his/her order of "no movement" and immediately start treating the horse with IV fluids and electrolytes to restore balance. Even though they're needed, he/she would resist the temptation to give additional medications, such as

- acepromazine to dilate the muscles' constricted blood vessels
- diuretics to help keep the kidneys working, and
- antiinflammatory medications like Banamine™, phenylbutazone ("bute"), or Ketofen™ to relieve the pain, spasms, and toxic effects,

until the fluids and electrolytes have had a chance to take effect. If given too soon to a horse in severely compromised condition, these medications can have dangerous side-effects that might even make the horse's condition worse. And even when it's safe to give them, the sharp veterinarian will give "light" doses — sometimes less than 1/3 the usual dose — to avoid adverse reactions.

Days (and sometimes weeks) later, after all the medications have been given and the pain is gone, the blood vessels in the muscles have relaxed, the urine's color is back to normal, and blood is again circulating properly through the muscles, he/she will give the go-ahead for slow, in-hand walking.

SPECIAL NOTE 12.1

Heart rates above 60 beats/min after at least 30 minutes of rest can indicate exhaustion and a toxic condition from muscle sickness. See *Chapter 13*.

TYPE B

If the diagnosis is Type B, the vet would order slow walking and muscle massage, usually within just a few hours after treatment for the underlying fluid, electrolyte, and fatigue problems. Why let the horse walk? Because unless the case is extremely severe and/or advanced, the muscles aren't dying— they're just "sick" from not getting the circulation they need. Once the constricted blood vessels have been coaxed into re-opening, the movement of slow walking will help to restore the circulation, get the muscle fibers sliding smoothly, and hasten recovery. Again, the administration of any medications for pain relief, vasodilation, and diuresis would be delayed until the fluid and electrolyte imbalances had been addressed and the horse had begun to show some signs of relief. With Type B myositis, the horse is often walking within an hour.

There's no vet. What should you do?

This is a common problem for endurance race competitors who take their horses on long training runs in the back country and for all horse people who, in addition to their equine passions, also have a day job that keeps them from riding every day and forces their horses to be weekend warriors. Those who are fortunate enough to live in an area where they can train "out the back door" have the luxury of familiar veterinary care as close as their kitchen telephone. But most have to trailer their horses some distance to find the right combination of miles and terrain — and when muscle disorders strike, a cool head and a good education are essential. Before you do anything, first take the following mini-test.

Figure out which type of muscle disorder your horse has. Check the answers that are true for his current situation and add up the scores to see which category he fits:

He's a high-strung animal.	If yes: add 1.
He was excited or anxious today.	If yes: add 1.
His muscle problem came on suddenly.	If yes: add 2.
His muscle problem showed up early, shortly after the start of exercise, before he really had a chance to get warmed up.	If yes: add 3.
"He's" a female, and she's young.	If yes: add 1.
He's had this problem before.	If yes: add 1.

If his score is 6 or higher, the odds are high that he has Type A myositis. If his score is 5 or below, he probably has Type B myositis.

Okay — you've got a tentative diagnosis. Here's what you should do:

SPECIAL NOTE 12.2

Don't have any commercial equine electrolytes? No problem — you can make your own with common grocery-store items. See *Chapter 13*.

Take this mini-test to determine whether your horse is stricken with Type A or Type B myositis.

STEP 1.
Freeze!

Do not move the Type A-stricken horse or you will only make him worse — he'll have to stay put for several days (and by then, you'll have a veterinarian to help you). Make him as comfortable as you can right where he is — if possible, "build" a makeshift stall around him, provide him with shelter from the elements, and attend to his problems where he stands. If he's lying down (less than 3% of cases do), give him soft bedding to protect his muscles from hard surfaces.

Do not move the Type B-stricken horse either, at least for the next hour or so, until you've had a chance to attend to some of his problems in the following steps.

STEP 2.
Check the T-P-R

Check temperature, pulse, and respiratory rate at least every half hour, and write them down — they'll tell you how your horse is responding and, if he's a Type B case, whether it's time to relax a bit and move him.

It's acceptable for a horse's temperature to rise to as high as 103º F with a good workout, but if it's a "normal fever," it should be accompanied by sweating and the temperature should come down, on its own, by at least one degree every 15 minutes. Once it gets down to 101º F, the sweating should subside.

If your horse's temperature is above 102º, *do not* run cold hose water over his major muscles to cool him — this might worsen the already dangerous constriction of blood vessels in those beleaguered muscles. Instead, put cool wet compresses on the side of his neck, behind his ears, and in his armpits, shelter him from the hot sun, and let the evaporation of his own sweat cool him off.

As soon as your examinations show you that the T-P-R readings are coming back down toward normal (temp approaching 101º F, pulse approaching 60 beats/min, respiratory rate approaching 18 breaths/min) the horse is eating and drinking willingly, and, if you happen to be watching when he urinates, it's not brown colored, then it's okay to start walking him at a relaxed rate (slow enough to stop once in a while and nibble or sniff). Don't be surprised if the urine is a very concentrated yellow — that's to be expected. You just don't want to move him unnecessarily if it's brown.

STEP 3.
Food and drink

Help your horse replenish his fluid and electrolyte losses, which are considerable after a long, hard, sweaty workout. Offer small handfuls of grass hay and sips of cool (NOT COLD!) water in half-gallon volumes at first, so he doesn't guzzle and upset his stomach or, horrors, cause laminitis. Bring the hay and water to him, don't make him walk for it. Alongside the bucket of plain water, at the same time offer a second bucket of electrolyte-treated water. IMPORTANT: Before you give your horse any electrolytes, read *Special Note 12.3*.

STEP 4.
Medicate

Medication in the field situation is reasonable only if your horse's case is severe and, as always, if your veterinarian has given you a prescription to use in just such a situation. Horses that have tied-up in the past are good candidates for this kind of protection, and if you've shown your vet that you understand how to use it properly,

SPECIAL NOTE 12.3

It's very important that you give the myositis-stricken horse the right kind of electrolytes. Give the wrong kind, and you can make his myositis much worse. Rule of thumb: read all labels.

Don't give the Type B myositis-stricken endurance horse an electrolyte preparation that contains sodium bicarbonate, especially if he's also showing signs of heat exhaustion (see *Chapter 13*). Look at the label for the words bicarb, bicarbonate, baking soda, sodium bicarbonate, or the chemical name $NaHCO_3$, and if you see any of these names on the label, don't give it — it'll definitely not produce the effect you're looking for. Electrolyte products made for calves and foals with diarrhea and for sprint-type equine athletes do contain sodium bicarbonate, which is often appropriate for those particular situations, but it's absolutely the wrong thing to give a horse with Type B myositis. If you have any doubt about what to give, don't give either commercial product — get the horse to replenish his debts by eating and drinking, or make your own electrolyte solution (see recipe on page 153). And be sure to always, always, offer a bucket of plain water at the same time.

SPECIAL NOTE 12.4

ASPIRIN DOSE FOR MYOSITIS:

800 lb horse:	3 grams
900 lb horse:	4 grams
1,000 lb horse:	4-1/2 grams
1,100 lb horse:	5 grams
1,200 lb horse:	5-1/2 grams
1,300 lb horse:	6 grams
1,400 lb horse:	6-1/2 grams

To be given orally, once only.

SPECIAL NOTE 12.5

BANAMINE™ DOSE FOR MYOSITIS:

800 lb horse:	2 cc
900 lb horse:	2 cc
1000 lb horse:	2-1/2 cc
1,100 lb horse:	2-1/2 cc
1,200 lb horse:	3 cc
1,300 lb horse:	3 cc
1,400 lb horse:	3 cc

To be given intramuscularly, once only.

SPECIAL NOTE 12.6

ACEPROMAZINE DOSE FOR MYOSITIS:

800 lb horse:	16 mg (=1.6 cc)
900 lb horse:	18 mg (=1.9 cc)
1,000 lb horse:	20 mg (=2 cc)
1,100 lb horse:	22 mg (=2.2 cc)
1,200 lb horse:	24 mg (=2.4 cc)
1,300 lb horse:	26 mg (=2.6 cc)
1,400 lb horse:	28 mg (=2.8 cc)

To be given intramuscularly, once only.

he/she may see an advance prescription for emergency relapses as a good idea. After he's willingly eaten and taken in some liquids, you'll know two things:

- first, that he's feeling well enough to eat, and
- second, that his system is benefiting from the moisture and natural electrolyte content of the feed he's consumed.

At this point, it's okay for the severely myositis-stricken patient to be given some medications to control the amount of damage done to his muscles. Mild cases won't need this treatment, nor will moderate cases if they were recognized and treated promptly. See *Special Notes #12.4, 12.5 and 12.6* for proper doses — the doses of these medications recommended for other conditions are likely to be too high for myositis.

a. Aspirin (paste, gel, or crushed tablets mixed in molasses and given orally) is the best choice for emergency field use because it requires no prescription and it's a remarkably effective drug for short-term relief of pain and longer-term blockage of the toxins that can amplify and prolong the damage of myositis. It is also an effective prostaglandin inhibitor, so it'll help to relax the blood vessels that have constricted in the muscles as a result of prostaglandin from tissue damage and toxins.

b. Banamine™ does the same things that aspirin does, but it's a bit more potent and long-lasting. Its use should be reserved for severe cases, and because of its potency, the warning about making sure the horse's hydration and electrolyte balance have improved before giving it should be given top priority. It is the most effective drug for blocking the action of the endotoxins, and it's also an impressive pain- and prostaglandin-fighter.

c. Acepromazine can help further dilate the blood vessels that have constricted in his muscles. Yes, it is a tranquilizer, but it's not the calming effect on your horse that we're looking for— it's the calming effect on his blood vessels. Again, this medication is warranted only in very severe cases, and since it's a prescription item, you'll have to have the prior blessing of your veterinarian.

STEP 5.
NO SELENIUM!!

Selenium is one of those "tightrope" medications: there's a very fine line between the amount the horse needs and the amount that will kill him.

Unless you've gotten prior approval from your veterinarian, *do not* treat a myositis-stricken horse with any of the many available vitamin E-selenium products. It's true that some cases of myositis have been attributed to a selenium deficiency, but if your horse doesn't need it (and most cases don't), you could create some real problems. Selenium is one of those "tightrope" minerals: the horse can't live without it, but there's a very fine line between the amount he needs and the amount that will kill him. Most horses get all the selenium they need in the hay and grass they eat. If your horse is deficient, it takes a blood test (about $20) and a bit of a wait (about a week) to find out. *Don't give the stuff unless you know he needs it.*

STEP 6.
Monitor his progress

Keep checking your horse's vital signs and his discomfort while making arrangements to secure a veterinarian's assessment. With any luck, even the most severe cases of muscle disorder will be stopped in their tracks by what you've done so far. Remember, it's important in the field situation to delay giving any medications until the horse has had a chance to get rehydrated and correct some of his electrolyte deficiencies. In the hospital setting, he'd undoubtedly be getting intravenous fluids for this problem, but in your case that's not possible. Don't jump the gun and medicate a badly dehydrated, electrolyte-deficient horse — wait until he's brightened, his T-P-R readings have shown real evidence of recovery, and his comfort level has improved. If it's a mild case, skip the meds — they aren't needed. If you're unsure, wait a while longer. It's difficult, but in the field situation you simply have to rely on judgment.

Should you seek veterinary assistance?

Absolutely, and as soon as possible, even if your horse recovers completely under your care. Even mild cases warrant a veterinary look-see because any information your horse provides might help pinpoint the cause of the problem and help you prevent it in the future, whether it's nutritional, genetic, a problem with temperament or the training program, or a combination. Remember, nearly 50% of all cases of myositis are repeat offenders. There's a statistic you'll want to beat!

CHAPTER 13

Heat Exhaustion

(also known as Exhausted Horse Syndrome)

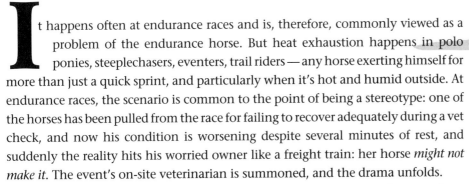

I t happens often at endurance races and is, therefore, commonly viewed as a problem of the endurance horse. But heat exhaustion happens in polo ponies, steeplechasers, eventers, trail riders — any horse exerting himself for more than just a quick sprint, and particularly when it's hot and humid outside. At endurance races, the scenario is common to the point of being a stereotype: one of the horses has been pulled from the race for failing to recover adequately during a vet check, and now his condition is worsening despite several minutes of rest, and suddenly the reality hits his worried owner like a freight train: her horse *might not make it*. The event's on-site veterinarian is summoned, and the drama unfolds.

But what if your horse is stricken and you're at an unsanctioned event, where there's no vet available? Or you're on a training run, rather than at an official event? Or it wasn't intentional exercise at all — your show horse somehow got out of his stall and has been running, terrified, with snarling dogs at his heels, for the past hour as the outside thermometer creeps up to 95º F and the relative humidity is close behind? What do you do?

What you see

The hallmark of advanced heat exhaustion is lack of interest in eating or drinking after a workout, despite the absolute certainty that, after the rigors of his exercise, the horse desperately needs the liquids and electrolytes that water and food would provide. The full list of signs includes:

- shortened stride, lack of impulsion
- elevated rectal temperature (as high as 104-107.6º F)
- depression, acts profoundly tired
- inattention: shows no interest in his surroundings
- unstable or persistently elevated heart rate
- persistently elevated respiratory rate, or panting
- the "thumps" (what appears to be a rhythmic jerking of the abdominal muscles with each breath, almost like violent hiccups)
- no appetite, no desire for water
- glazed look in the eyes
- "quiet gut" — the normal motility of the intestines has slowed
- sweat-soaked or, paradoxically, *less* than expected sweating
- scant and very concentrated urine

The goal in dealing with this dangerous condition is catching it in its earliest stages, before the diagnosis is obvious and before the horse's cardiovascular system breaks down.

What's going on inside

When an equine athlete's muscles are asked to do work, they generate two things: horsepower (to move the horse forward) and heat (which serves no purpose but is, rather, a by-product of exercise, like exhaust from an automobile's engine). As the work continues, the extra heat accumulates in the body, and body temperature rises.

In the endurance horse, the heat generated by the race's moderate-intensity, long-term demands is about 18 - 27 º F per hour — if all of that heat remained in his body, the horse would be a hard-boiled egg by the middle of the race.

But the horse stays relatively cool because he has four ways to help dissipate some of that heat:

1. some of it simply radiates from his body, like a hot brick wall radiates warmth into a home — an inefficient method for the horse;

2. it can be conducted away when his hot body leans against a cold surface, a technique that is much more important for hot dogs lying on cold floors than hot horses running in the sun;

3. some of it is carried away by convection on a cool breeze —again, not very efficient;

4. and most importantly for the horse, it is dissipated by evaporation — evaporation of sweat from his body, and evaporation of moisture from his breath. Evaporation is the horse's ace in the hole, with as much as two-thirds of the heat generated by exercise being eliminated by evaporating sweat, about one-fourth by evaporating moisture from his panting breath, and the rest being stored in the body

SPECIAL NOTE 13.1

Anhidrosis occurs most often in horses that live and work in hot, humid climates. Their chronically stimulated sweat glands are permanently "burned out."

to raise the mercury on the rectal thermometer. As long as his ability to dissipate heat via sweat and breath evaporation is working well, he should be able to escape heat exhaustion.

However, there are some factors that will foil his ability to cool himself by evaporation. The ability to sweat, for example, is less developed in horses that are inadequately conditioned. And as many as 20% of horses that have lived and competed in the Gulf Coast states are victims of a dangerous condition called *anhidrosis* — their sweat glands are literally worn out (see *Special Note 13.1*) and can no longer produce the sweat needed to safely cool themselves during a long workout.

Horses that begin an event already "hot" are also at a disadvantage — if they're nervous, for example, due to an anxious temperament or due to inexperience with the excitement of the event, or if they just got off the horse trailer after a long trip to the event (see *Special Note 13.2*).

And the biggest danger of all is the weather. When it's hot and humid outside, the horse's ability to sweat might be intact, but his sweat and respiratory moisture simply aren't going to *evaporate*, so he isn't going to be cooled (see *Special Note 13.3*).

To make matters worse, in a typical endurance competition a horse can sweat away as much as 12 gallons of water and electrolytes. In fact, the combined fluid loss from sweat, urine, feces, and the moisture in the breath can be as much as four gallons per hour during a race. This leads to dehydration and hypovolemia (low blood volume), making it harder for the body to perform in the ongoing competition, and making it much more difficult to compensate for accumulating heat.

In the horse, sweat is actually "richer" in the "salt" minerals (sodium, potassium, chloride, and magnesium) than the blood is. This means that when he becomes dehydrated because of massive sweating, he also becomes deficient in all the minerals he's losing in his sweat. He becomes deficient in calcium too, and this calcium debt can be so profound that it causes the "thumps," technically called *synchronous diaphragmatic flutter.* This is actually a rapid jerking of the diaphragm every time the heart beats (since the horse is breathing rapidly, it might appear that the jerking coincides with each *breath*, but it's actually linked to the pumping of the heart.) The phrenic nerve, which supplies electrical impulses to the diaphragm, reacts to the horse's electrolyte imbalance by becoming overly sensitive to being "bumped," and since it drapes over the heart on its way to the diaphragm, it gets bumped every time the heart beats. Every nudge stimulates the nerve to fire, which causes the diaphragm to jump, which gives the horse an eerie, herky-jerky abdominal "flinch" with every heart beat.

SPECIAL NOTE 13.2

The muscle activity needed to stand and balance during a long trailer ride raises the body temperature and can shorten the time it takes for the horse to heat up in the race.

SPECIAL NOTE 13.3

How hot and humid is too hot and humid? It varies with the horse's conditioning, his experience (is he acclimated to hot, humid weather?), the rigors of the event, and whether he's got anhidrosis (see *Special Note 13.1*), but here's the rule of thumb. Add the outside temperature, in degrees Fahrenheit, to the relative humidity: (example: 90° F and 79% relative humidity: 90 + 79 = 169). If the total is greater than 150, all competitors are at risk of heat exhaustion.

Why is heat exhaustion dangerous?

This is much more than just a bad case of fatigue. It's a dangerous buildup of heat in the horse's body which, if unresolved, can lead to cardiovascular instability, collapse, and death.

Right before your very eyes.

How does it happen?

The electrolyte deficits in the exhausted horse can be astounding, and since the sensation of thirst is linked to the detection of *excess* salt in the system, the salt-deficient horse feels no desire to drink. This means that, if left to his own devices, he would be unlikely to recover because despite his dehydration he has no natural urge to replace the liquids he so desperately needs.

To naturally replace electrolytes, the horse must eat. However, if his mineral deficiency is severe enough to cause his gut motility to slow down, he's got a belly ache — it might be very mild and subtle, or it might appear as full-blown colic — but even the mildest colic pain can squelch his desire to eat. He *must* eat, but he *won't*.

Meanwhile, he continues to pant in an attempt to blow off the heat that is killing him from the inside. But with each breath he can become more dehydrated, and the muscular activity involved in panting can actually stoke the fire, creating more heat.

As his cardiovascular system collapses, blood vessels to the muscles and skin begin to constrict closed. This keeps his too-hot blood close to his core, away from the body's surface where it had the best chance of dissipating its extra heat. It also sets the horse up for myositis (tying-up; see *Chapter 12*), because those muscles, which are sorely in need of nourishment after their workout, are suddenly being cut off.

At the very least, the horse's career is at stake.

But to be brutally blunt, the victim of exhausted horse syndrome is at risk of collapsing and dying.

What would the vet do?

The horse's problems are twofold: he's way too hot, and he's got a serious deficiency of water and electrolytes. The other things — the "thumping," the rapid heart rate, the abdominal pain, the depression — they're all secondary symptoms. Therefore, the experienced veterinarian should focus on getting the horse cooled, getting him rehydrated, and taking care of his electrolyte deficiencies first. Then, and only then, will he give medications for those secondary problems, and in many cases they'll be resolving on their own, thanks to the attention given to the primary problems.

Because the horse continues to pant and sweat, even after being withdrawn from the race, treatment must focus on stopping any further loss of fluid and electrolytes as well as replacing those already lost. By placing an intravenous catheter in the horse's jugular vein, the vet can begin administering fluids containing the

This is much more than just a bad case of fatigue. It's a dangerous buildup of heat in the horse's body which, if unresolved, can lead to cardiovascular instability, collapse, and death.

With each panting breath he can become more dehydrated, and the muscular activity involved in that heavy breathing can actually stoke his internal fire, creating even more heat.

electrolytes that are most deficient — it's not uncommon to give as much as ten gallons of IV fluids over the first few hours of treatment. A commercial IV product containing glucose, calcium, and magnesium (calcium borogluconate) can be included in the IV fluids if the horse's condition is severe enough to show signs of "thumps," but the vet will have to keep a stethoscope on the heart to listen for signs of adverse reaction to the calcium (give it too fast, and the heart can become erratic or simply stop).

While the fluids are being given, effort should be made to cool the horse's innards by assisting the evaporative cooling process: providing an electric fan if there's no breeze, carefully giving frequent cool (not cold) water rinses, rigging up some shade, standing the horse in a shallow pool.

Even if the horse is showing overt signs of colic, the sharp veterinarian will not give any medication for abdominal pain until a significant dose of IV fluids and electrolytes has been given — in his fragile state, the exhausted horse can easily have a fatal reaction to *any* medications. Furthermore, as the fluids and electrolytes begin to restore gut function, accumulated gases begin to move along and the colic pain should subside.

In his fragile state, the exhausted horse can have a fatal reaction to any medications.

Once the horse begins to show signs of improvement, the vet will give a nonsteroidal antiinflammatory drug (such as Banamine™ or "bute") to block the destruction of muscle tissue from inflammation, to protect the horse from toxins, and to make him more comfortable so he'll eat and drink more readily. He might also give a vasoactive drug (such as acepromazine) to dilate the blood vessels that had begun to constrict in the horse's muscles, hopefully to ward off myositis.

Throughout treatment, small amounts of feed, cool (not cold), plain water, and electrolyte-treated water should be offered to the patient as his condition improves and he regains the desire to replace his losses orally.

There's no vet. What should you do?

Horses that are stricken with heat exhaustion while performing some shorter-term, high-intensity exercise such as 3-day eventing or polo are likely to have less critical need for fluids and are simply in need of help in lowering their core temperatures. For these horses, repeated cool (not cold) water baths and slow, relaxed walking in a light breeze is likely to do the trick. Getting the horse to eat and drink is rarely a challenge, so he'll probably replenish his fluids and electrolytes on his own.

Early in the course of heat exhaustion, the horse might appear bright and normal, but he needs to be pushed to keep up the pace, and if you checked his rectal temperature it might be as high as 104º F. Treatment at this point would be simple and effective. An hour later, when his distress is obvious, treating him would be much more "touch and go."

The endurance horse is a different case — his fluid and electrolyte debts are likely to be astounding and possibly life-threatening, and without the option of administering intravenous fluids and electrolytes, you're severely limited. However, even though you're in serious trouble in this situation and should move heaven and earth to get a competent equine veterinarian to come to your aid, you should still be able to help the horse if you're prepared. Ready? Let's get started.

STEP 1.
Check vitals

Check the rectal temperature, the number of heart beats per minute, the number of breaths per minute, and listen to the abdomen for gut sounds (see *Chapter 19: Vital Signs*, for proper procedure), and write all your findings down. Re-check every half hour and record your progress.

STEP 2.
Electrolytes and Fluids

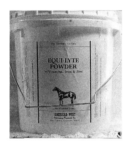

Gently but persistently get electrolytes and fluids into the horse orally. If he won't eat or drink voluntarily, you'll have to use some initiative to coax him.

Suggestions:

■ Offer a bucket containing a half gallon of plain, cool (not cold) water and, right next to it, a second bucket containing a half gallon of electrolyte-treated water using a commercially prepared electrolyte powder designed specifically for endurance horses. Do not, under any circumstances, give this horse an electrolyte product made for calves or foals with scours (diarrhea) or for sprinting-activity performance horses — the sodium bicarbonate in these products can make his heart unstable, and it can guarantee that he will be stricken with myositis on top of all his other problems (see *Special Note 13.4*).

■ If he shows no interest in trying either bucket, rinse his mouth gently with a 20 cc syringe full of the electrolyte-treated water, then offer the buckets again.

■ Still no luck? Try squirting a teaspoon (five cc) of Karo™ syrup (corn syrup), honey, molasses, or a thick paste of sugar and water into his mouth, wait a few minutes, then offer the buckets again.

■ Still no luck? You'll have to force him. Remember, he's still losing more water and electrolytes, probably a gallon or more per hour, even though he's just standing there — they're literally pouring out of him in his sweat and in his breath.

Start with the electrolytes first. Read the instructions on the label of your electrolyte product and calculate how much of the product would be required to prepare one quart of treated water.

Example: If the instructions say to add a "scoop" of their product to four gallons of water, measure out how many teaspoons are in the scoop they include in the package. Let's say the scoop holds 16 teaspoons. There are 16 quarts in four gallons, so each quart should have one teaspoon of product. (The amount may be different for your particular product).

Mix the calculated amount of product in 1/2 cup of something smooth and yummy, such as canned baby food (Gerber's oatmeal with applesauce, pureed carrots, pears, and vanilla pudding are popular choices). If it's not a naturally sweet product, add a couple tablespoons of honey, Karo syrup, sugar, or molasses. Don't have any baby food? That's okay, use your imagination to make a concoction with other items that are logical for horses (instant oatmeal, applesauce, carrot juice, apple butter, molasses, etc.) — the idea is to mix a quart's worth of electrolyte product into a sweet,

---

SPECIAL NOTE 13.4

Be sure to give the heat-exhaustion-stricken horse the right kind of electrolytes. Give the wrong kind, and you can cause myositis and maybe even a heart attack. Rule of thumb: read all labels. Never, ever give the heat-exhaustion endurance victim any products that contain sodium bicarbonate (a.k.a. "bicarb," "baking soda," "soda," "bicarbonate of soda," or "NaHCO$_3$"). Electrolyte products made for calves with diarrhea, and for sprint-type horse athletes, often contain sodium bicarbonate — it's appropriate for them. But in your endurance horse, use only what was made for endurance horses.

tasty gruel with a consistency that can be squeezed into the horse's mouth with an empty paste-dewormer syringe.

Give him your concoction with the syringe and let him work it around in his mouth, taste how good it is, and swallow most of it.

Now squirt two cups of water, by several syringefuls, into his mouth to help him wash it all down, and wait ten minutes.

Offer the buckets again, as well as a handful of grass hay.

Still no luck? Okay, you'll have to get more aggressive. Give him one cup of water, by syringe, every five minutes, and give another dose of electrolyte gruel, by syringe, every half hour (see *Special Note 13.5*). Do this for two hours, or until he begins drinking on his own, whichever comes first.

Don't have any electrolyte powder? Well, okay, you can make your own concoction with ingredients you can buy at any grocery store in the spice section, the tummy ache section, the vitamin-mineral-pharmacy section, and the baking supplies section. Be sure to get enough supplies to give several doses — you might have to treat your horse for a few hours before he begins to respond.

1 Tablespoon regular table salt (sodium chloride)

1 Tablespoon Morton's salt substitute (potassium chloride)

2 crushed tablets of extra-strength TUMS™ (calcium carbonate)

500 mg (2 crushed 250-mg tablets) of magnesium pills (magnesium oxide)

2 Tablespoons Karo syrup or honey or molasses or pancake syrup

1 jar of Gerber's baby food (some horse-appropriate flavor)

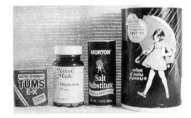

Meanwhile, be working on bringing his body temperature down by swabbing him every ten minutes with cool (not cold), dripping-wet cloths over his body, being sure to get him behind and between his ears, on his forehead, on the underside of his neck, and in his armpits and groin. Do not run *cold* hose water over his back and rump — you could cause the blood vessels in those muscles to clamp closed even more than they already are, which will slow down his heat dissipation and threaten myositis.

As soon as you see signs of improvement: a brighter look in the eye, heart rate beginning to drop to within normal range, respiratory panting beginning to resolve, body temperature coming back down to earth, and a return to voluntary eating and drinking, give a tiny, *tiny* dose of aspirin paste or gel orally to relieve residual muscle pain, encourage the still-spasming muscles to relax, and guard against the damaging effects of inflammation and endotoxemia. If you have no aspirin, but your vet entrusted you with an emergency dose of Banamine™, you'll have to decide whether the horse is in good enough shape to tolerate medication. Rule of thumb: don't risk it. But if you can't seem to get him comfortable, or you think he might be developing

SPECIAL NOTE 13.5

Be careful not to force oral liquids too quickly, or some of the water might go "down the wrong tube." Squirt the water in the space between cheek and side teeth, without forcing the syringe between his teeth, and hold his chin just high enough to cause the water to roll toward the back of his throat.

STEP 3.
Cool him

STEP 4.
Give aspirin

myositis, and you've gotten at least two doses of electrolytes into him, you may have nothing to lose. Whatever you decide, use the doses given in *Special Notes 13.6 and 13.7* — the doses recommended for other conditions are likely to be way too high.

STEP 5.
What about his muscles?

If your horse is showing any signs of impending myositis (stiffening gait, tight or hard-feeling muscles over his back, croup, and loins, and/or coffee-colored urine), or if he has a history of tying-up in the past, he might benefit from a judicial dose of acepromazine to dilate the constricted blood vessels in his major muscles (see *Special Note 13.8*). Again, if he's in very tough shape, he might not be able to tolerate any medication smoothly, and if you give anything indiscriminantly you could be taking a huge chance. If your vet thinks you're savvy enough about such things that he/she has entrusted you with some acepromazine for emergency situations, you're probably able to assess your horse's condition and decide whether or not it's worth the risk. Rule of thumb: if he's eating and drinking well on his own, and he seems to be showing general signs of recovery, he should be able to tolerate this medication.

STEP 6.
Set up camp

If you're far from home, it's really better to set up camp where you are, rather than trailer the horse a long distance. Similarly, if the nearest vet is a long trailer ride away, you'd be better off bribing him/her to drive to wherever you are. Why? The muscular work involved in standing and balancing in a horse trailer is almost universally underestimated. Trust me, it's *substantial*. If your horse suffered a serious bout of exhaustion and, during the 12-24 hours afterwards you load him up and trailer him, the muscle exertion he'll have to expend in order to stay on his feet in the trailer can cause him to develop myositis or, if he's already got myositis, his beleaguered muscles might be seriously damaged by working to stabilize him in the trailer, and the fragments of pulverized muscle cells will threaten to damage his kidneys.

SPECIAL NOTE 13.6 ASPIRIN DOSE: HEAT EXHAUSTION		SPECIAL NOTE 13.7 BANAMINE™ DOSE: HEAT EXHAUSTION		SPECIAL NOTE 13.8 ACEPROMAZINE DOSE	
800 lb horse:	1-1/2 grams	800 lb horse:	1-1/2 cc	800 lb horse:	16 mg (=1.6 cc)
900 lb horse:	2 grams	900 lb horse:	1-3/4 cc	900 lb horse:	18 mg (=1.9 cc)
1,000 lb horse:	2 grams	1,000 lb horse:	2 cc	1,000 lb horse:	20 mg (=2 cc)
1,100 lb horse:	2-1/2 grams	1,100 lb horse:	2 cc	1,100 lb horse:	22 mg (=2.2cc)
1,200 lb horse:	2-1/2 grams	1,200 lb horse:	2-1/2 cc	1,200 lb horse:	24 mg (=2.4cc)
1,300 lb horse:	3 grams	1,300 lb horse:	2-1/2 cc	1,300 lb horse:	26 mg (=2.6cc)
1,400 lb horse:	3 grams	1,400 lb horse:	3 cc	1,400 lb horse:	28 mg (=2.8cc)
To be given orally, once only.		To be given intramuscularly, once only.		To be given intramuscularly, once only.	

CHAPTER 14

Respiratory Disease

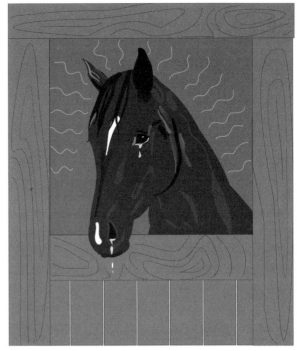

I t's small wonder that respiratory disease is the most common malady that
afflicts the performance horse. After all, look at his environment: dusty/
moldy bedding, dusty hay, dusty oats, dusty arenas, dusty rides in trailers
behind fume-y towing vehicles, stalls and trailers deeply marinated in the bracing
aroma of ammonia, and exposure to lots of other horses that might not be as healthy,
well vaccinated, religiously dewormed, and compulsively protected as yours is. And
the performance horse's stressful, high-anxiety lifestyle makes him even more of a
target.

Still, your performer is well protected: he's healthy, well conditioned, a
seasoned competitor, and he's vaccinated against every condition for which there's
a vaccine. So when fever, runny nose, and/or cough strike him en route to or from
a competition, you react with a mixture of alarm and frustration. Where did he catch
it? How long will he be out of circulation? He *will* be okay, won't he? The answers
might surprise you.

What you see

It'll vary with the source of your horse's ailment, but he'll select his symptoms from
the following list:

- harsh, dry cough; or soft, juicy cough
- fever
- loss of appetite
- depression
- stiff, sore muscles

- watery eyes
- watery, runny nasal discharge; or snotty, thicker nasal discharge
- swelling of the legs
- enlargement of the "glands" under the jaw
- rapid, shallow "panting"
- exquisitely tender chest wall

What's going on inside

The most dangerous respiratory diseases are usually caused by "normal" germs from the horse's own mouth.

The horse's respiratory tract is remarkably well armed to protect it against the barrage of insults it endures in the typical performance horse's life. The "upper" respiratory tract (the nasal passages, the windpipe [trachea], and its two largest branches [bronchi]) are equipped with glands that secrete a tacky mucus that acts as a natural "fly paper" to catch and hold debris and infectious microorganisms before they make their way down to the lungs (the "lower" respiratory tract). Once trapped, the invaders are escorted out of the system by gravity (when the horse lowers his head to graze, the mucus and its prisoners drain out onto the ground), and by the rhythmic, dance-like beating of tiny hairlike cilia that line the windpipe and bronchi, setting up a sort of slow current to help sweep the bug-embedded mucus out.

In some cases, respiratory disease results when your horse simply becomes overwhelmed immunologically, as when he's exposed to some wicked germ that side-steps his vaccination program. It's no different for ourselves: when trapped in an elevator with some gushing, sneezing, germ-spewing victim of the common cold, we just don't stand a chance, no matter how well we take care of ourselves.

The horse's natural response to a respiratory infection is a self-defeating allergic-type reaction that almost always makes the situation worse — it allows the infecting organism to create the "best" (worst) symptoms it can.

In many of the most dangerous cases, however, respiratory disease comes from the horse's own baggage — from the germs and irritants in his immediate environment, and, surprisingly enough, *from his own mouth.*

That's right — the life-threatening cases of "shipping fever" and pneumonia are most often the result of "normal" germs from the horse's mouth taking advantage of a management slip-up that interfered with his natural defenses.

Slip-ups such as tying a trailering horse's head too short, so he can't drop it low enough during the trip to allow the bug-laden mucus to drain out of his upper respiratory tract.

Slip-ups such as letting him get dehydrated during the trip, which makes that mucus fly-paper too thick to drain properly.

Slip-ups such as thoughtfully (but unwisely) closing up the trailer windows when the weather turns nasty so your steed stays warm and dry, rather than leaving them open to keep the ammonia fumes from accumulating and irritating his respiratory lining.

Innocent, easy mistakes that take a situation that's pregnant with disease possibilities and turn those possibilities into reality. All the "bug" needs to do to win its quest is to find a way to hang around in the respiratory tract long enough to become established there.

For the most part, the horse's first lines of defense are very effective. But once a pathogen gets past them, it burrows in and starts reproducing. At this point, infection is no longer a possibility — it's a fact.

The body reacts to the infection by creating a condition called *airway hyperresponsiveness* — this is a self-defeating, allergic-type reaction that causes the muscles in the tube-like airways to squeeze down and make them suffocatingly narrow. This makes it difficult for the horse to breathe, which creates anxiety: more stress.

To make matters worse, the presence of the infecting organism in the tissues causes inflammation—heat, swelling, pain, and redness—which narrows them even further. Specialized cells whose job is to perpetuate inflammation infiltrate the respiratory tract and cause erosion of the system's lining, allowing even more bugs to gain entrance — this is the immune system's puzzling tendency to throw open the barn doors after the bull got out, as though letting all the other livestock loose will somehow help the situation. Which, of course, it doesn't — it allows bacteria to move in and set up secondary infections in horses already down with a viral infection.

The narrowed airways create even more inflammation because it's harder to squeeze air through them — whereas the normal airway is like a wide, calm, slow-moving river, the narrowed airway is like a roiling, boiling whitewater passageway, and the churning rush through that narrow passageway carves and scrapes at the walls with increased friction. Tissues that are already inflamed are being physically irritated even more, just from the process of pulling turbulent air through them.

The final blow that keeps inflammation burning in the infected respiratory tract is the secretion of caustic chemicals called *prostaglandins*. The presence of these chemicals in the beleaguered respiratory tract causes more contraction of the airway muscles (making it more difficult to get air into the lungs), constriction of the blood vessels around the airways (making it more difficult to get oxygen into the blood), more mucus secretion (clogging up already narrowed airways), and more damage to the system's lining (causing even more inflammation). The worse it gets, the worse it gets.

So, respiratory infection in the horse is an inflammmatory, suffocating, miserable proposition, no matter what the cause, and the length of time it takes to restore the respiratory tract to its previous state of good health is much greater than is traditionally believed. Even when it's just a self-limiting, viral, upper respiratory "cold," the effect on a performance horse's career can be considerable, particularly when the competitive season is relatively short.

By the way: the respiratory tract's highly irritable state ("hyperresponsiveness") persists for 4 -8 weeks after recovery from the infection, something you should bear in mind before sending your horse back to work.

In a recent study, 64% of all adult horses hospitalized for pneumonia had a history of recent trailer transport. Does your trailering technique threaten your horse's respiratory health?

What would the vet do?

Figuring out whether the infection is viral or bacterial is usually a process of educated guesswork. The sharp veterinarian will consider not only the horse's symptoms but also his circumstances:

- are there other horses in the vicinity showing signs of the same infection?
- was this horse recently trailered a long distance?
- was his recent trailering experience hampered by any of the aforementioned "slip-ups?"
- what's his vaccination status?

THE MOST COMMON DIAGNOSES

A. The Viral "Cold"

If a respiratory infection seems to be "going around," odds are your horse's ailment is viral, it's upper respiratory (infecting the trachea and bronchi, rather than the lungs), and it's probably due to one of the three most common viral respiratory bugs (influenza, "rhino" [equine rhinopneumonitis], or EVA [equine viral arteritis]). The symptoms are usually a combination of dry, harsh cough, fever, muscle stiffness, thin watery nasal discharge, and lack of appetite. EVA has the added attraction of causing edema in the legs. To everyone's frustration, flu and rhino can even affect horses that are vaccinated, because they can develop minor variations that side-step the protection given by the vaccines. (But that's not a good reason to stop vaccinating — unvaccinated horses are usually hit harder than those that have some, albeit only partial, protection from vaccination.)

B. Strangles

Strangles is a bacterial infection that can cause a multi-victim outbreak of upper respiratory disease. The vet probably won't have any trouble distinguishing Strangles from a viral infection because its symptoms are usually pretty unique: profound sore throat, soft juicy cough, and massively swollen "glands" under the jaw, in addition to the generic signs of fever, runny nose and poor appetite.

C. Pneumonia and Pleuropneumonia ("shipping fever")

If the horse was recently trailered a long distance, and if his trailering experience included human-induced management errors that magnified the insults to his respiratory tract and hampered his ability to sweep bugs and junk out of it, the odds are increased that he's got pleuropneumonia, a bacterial infection of the lungs and the Saran-wrap-like membrane that surrounds the lungs (the pleura). People tend to think bacterial infections are "less bad" than viral infections because we have antibiotics to fight bacteria, while we are powerless to fight viruses. But the truth is, pleuropneumonia is the deadliest respiratory infection an adult horse can get, killing as many as a third of its victims. If treatment is delayed or otherwise inappropriate, and sometimes even if everything is done absolutely right, pleuropneumonia can be devastating.

Treatment for viral infections is generally a matter of "riding it out," keeping the horse comfortable and keeping the fever low enough (around 101º F) so that he'll continue eating and drinking, and giving the nonsteroidal antiinflammatory drug Banamine™ to block the action of the inflammatory prostaglandins that are trying to perpetuate the fire in his upper respiratory system. Whether or not antibiotics are given is a judgment call — obviously they aren't going to do a thing to the viruses in the horse's system, but they might be able to fight a secondary bacterial infection. Trouble is, if the secondary bacterial infection hasn't started yet, giving antibiotics might simply fight off the bacteria that are sensitive to that antibiotic and pave the way for a tougher bacterium to move in, one against which we might not have an effective antibiotic. It's a tough call, one that should not be made flippantly.

Treatment for Strangles is similar to that for viral infections, but the enlarged "glands" (lymph nodes) under the jaw might also need to be lanced and drained. The bacterial cause of Strangles is vulnerable to antibiotics, but the vet will have to exercise judgment in deciding whether or not to administer antibiotics because the wrong drug, the wrong dose, or the wrong timing can cause the bug to move out of the upper respiratory tract and into the bloodstream, where it can coast along until it finds a "better" place to set up housekeeping (like the liver, or the brain, or in scattered abscesses throughout the body). It's called "bastard Strangles," and it's nothing to toy with.

If the vet suspects pleuropneumonia, further diagnostic tests will be done to see if pus has accumulated between the lungs and the pleura, using ultrasound and x-rays. In many cases, there are *gallons* of pus, and treatment has to be somewhat radical in order to be successful — drains must be surgically installed to get the pus out so the horse can breathe, high doses of expensive antibiotics are given intravenously, and in some cases the horse must be supported in an intensive care unit. Quarantine is usually not warranted, because pleuropneumonia is not really that contagious — the horse fell victim to the condition because of a conspiracy of circumstances, rather than exposure to some virulent bug, and in most cases the bug is a normal inhabitant of every horse's mouth that simply got the opportunity to invade the respiratory tract and decided to go for it.

There's no vet. What should you do?

First and foremost, withdraw the horse from competition and isolate him from other horses, both to protect them from catching something from him and to protect him from catching something more from them. Regardless of whether his infection involves the upper or the lower respiratory tract, regardless of whether it's viral or bacterial, and regardless of whether it's a dangerous condition or just an annoying bout with the equine equivalent of the "common cold," the stress, exertion, and heavy breathing associated with performance are guaranteed to make a mountain out

Because bacteria can be killed with antibiotics, while there's nothing to kill viruses, people tend to believe that bacterial infections are "better" than viral infections. Wrong. The deadliest respiratory infection of adult horses is bacterial pleuropneumonia.

Pleuropneumonia is not particularly contagious — the bug is usually a normal inhabitant of every horse's mouth that got the opportunity to invade the respiratory tract and decided to go for it.

STEP 1.
Withdraw and isolate

of what might have started out as a molehill. Don't risk it — *forget* the event and focus on your horse.

STEP 2.
Check the vitals

Collect data on his current condition by taking his temperature, counting how many breaths he takes per minute when at rest, counting the number of heartbeats per minute at rest, looking for watery or thick nasal discharge, checking his appetite (offer just a little of his favorite thing and see if he's interested), and checking to see if his ribcage is sore to being gently but firmly pressed with your fingertips. Write all this information down and update it regularly. The most often re-checked items should be his temperature, his respiratory rate, and his appetite — get new readings, and write them down, every hour so you can see if your treatment is helping him.

If he shows signs of resentment or pain when you press gently on his ribcage, it's beginning to look like pleuropneumonia.

STEP 3.
Provide a pure environment

Place him in an environment that is absolutely not going to make his situation worse. The ideal would be an outdoor, open-air paddock that is shielded from bad weather but that has none of the ventilation hazards that a stall would have. If it's cold out, you can blanket him rather than put him inside. Ammonia fumes from urine-soaked bedding are one of the most potent irritators of the respiratory tract, and dust and mold spores from bedding are another. Therefore, the best thing to give him for bedding would be clean, soft grass. An added advantage of the grassy paddock is that the horse will lower his head to graze, which will help drain out the mucus that is becoming trapped in his narrowing upper respiratory airways. If a grassy bed is not possible, use something with little or no dust, such as shredded paper, rice hulls, or wood shavings rather than straw, hay, or sawdust. Don't be fooled into thinking that you can improve dusty bedding by wetting it down — all you'll do is stimulate the bedding's resident mold spores to wake up and join the party. And be compulsive about keeping his area meticulously clean — pick up all manure and dig out all urine before it affects air quality.

STEP 4.
Deal with the fever

Fever plays a role in fighting off infection by turning up the heat to a level that the infectious organism finds difficult to multiply in. However, like so many other responses of the equine body, fever can get out of control and create more problems than it solves (such as dehydration and excessive respiratory inflammation). The appetite is lousy when there's a fever, and the feverish horse will be unlikely to eat or drink enough to keep himself adequately hydrated. This is made worse by the fact that the fever causes him to breathe more rapidly, so he "blows off" more than the usual amount of moisture in his breath, bringing dehydration on even faster.

If he's drinking less than his usual amount of water, and/or if his fever is 103º F or greater, immediately take steps to bring it down to about 101º F. Your choices are

- **PHYSICAL** (rubdowns with isopropyl alcohol every half hour, cool water baths every half hour, and/or ice water-soaked towels frequently swabbed over the forehead, behind the ears, and in the armpits every 15 minutes), or

- **CHEMICAL** (aspirin paste or gel orally or, if you have it, an intramuscular injection of Banamine™ — see *Special Notes 14.3 and 14.4* for doses).

For horses with fevers in the 101-103º F range, the physical fever-fighting strategy is probably most appropriate, as long as the horse's appetite and water-drinking return when the fever comes down. For horses with higher fevers, or for lower fevers that aren't responding to external cooling attempts, go to the chemical weapon (see *Special Note 14.2*).

Aspirin requires no prescription and is a very effective fever fighter as well as a good antidote for those caustic prostaglandins that are perpetuating the inflammation.

But the higher the fever, the greater is the need for "the big gun": **Banamine™**. It should bring the fever down by several degrees within an hour, and it's the most effective anti-prostaglandin agent available. If your veterinarian gave you a dose of Banamine™ for emergency use, now's the time to use it. If not, use aspirin.

Stress, including the stress of a trailer ride, is the last thing this horse needs right now. Even if you tie him loosely so he can lower his head in the trailer, he's unlikely to take advantage of that in his current state. Another problem: the muscular exertion required to stand and balance in a moving horse trailer is universally underestimated — it's a significant physical stress that should be avoided if at all possible. And now that he's sick, the weather works against him whether it's pleasant or crummy — cold and damp weather will only stress him more, but if you close up the trailer to keep him warm and dry you'll shut down the ventilation; and if it's dry and warm outside, odds are that the trip will kick all sorts of dust and debris into the trailer to irritate his respiratory system even more. If you're at a facility that can easily be adapted to a "hospital sick room" function, you're better off bringing an equine vet to the horse. If, however, your setup is hopelessly primitive where intensive care for a pleuropneumonia victim would be impossible, you have no choice but to trailer him. In that case, do the preliminary work before loading him: find the vet, arrange for him/her to meet you at the hospital, figure out the best route to take, make sure the trailer is clean and fresh-smelling, blanket the horse to protect him from drafts, and drive with the windows open for ventilation.

SPECIAL NOTE 14.1

Normal temp:
99-100.5º F

Normal heart rate:
36-44 beats/min

Normal resp rate:
12-14 breaths/min

Expect all three to be elevated in the horse with a respiratory disease:

elev. temp: 101-106º F
elev. heart rate: 46-80 beats/min
elev. resp. rate: 16-40 breaths/min

STEP 5.
Stay put, if possible

SPECIAL NOTE 14.2

Important caveat:
Aspirin and Banamine™ can have serious side-effects (gastrointestinal ulcers) if used repeatedly in horses that are dehydrated and not eating normally. If you must use a drug to bring the fever down, choose only *one*, and use it only once.

STEP 6.
Heads down

Rather than use hay racks or nets, clean a spot on the ground (or lay a clean, smooth piece of plywood or a canvas drop cloth on the ground) and put the hay there, so the horse's head will be lowered as much as possible. Likewise, if his water bucket is in a wall-mounted holder, take it out and place it on the ground.

STEP 7.
No antibiotics
No antihistamines
No cough suppressants

It's not a good idea to give any of these drugs.

There is no antibiotic that is appropriate for all respiratory infections, despite the universal tendency of some people to give the same antibiotic for seemingly every malady. The selection of organisms that could be causing your horse's infection is immense, and what might be just the ticket for one bug might be the wrong choice for another. Without diagnostic laboratory tests, you have no way of knowing what bug you're treating, and there's a very real possibility that you'll be making a bad situation worse.

Antihistamines might make sense in theory, but they'll significantly thicken and dry the mucus in the upper respiratory tract to the point where it can't drain, and the waving cilia will be paralyzed in the stiff goo. As a result, the mucus will just stick to the respiratory walls and add to the horse's misery.

Cough suppressants might make *you* feel better, but that cough is important for kicking out the thick mucus and pus in the respiratory tree. All that muck will just keep accumulating if you suppress the cough.

Instead, focus your efforts on keeping the horse comfortable and hydrated, protecting him against the ravages of inflammation, and finding veterinary help if you have any suspicion of pneumonia.

Should you seek veterinary assistance?

If the whole barn is full of coughing, sneezing horses, and you're doing pretty well keeping your horse comfortable and hydrated, you can probably forego the veterinary call — there's not much the vet can do except tell you what you already know: your horse has a viral upper respiratory infection. Give the horse a lot of attention and pampering, frequent fresh water changes, brushing, coaxing him to eat and keep hydrated — all the nursing you'd crave if you were ill. Figure on at least three weeks before *slowly, gradually* beginning to return to work. He should not be back to his full work schedule until four to eight weeks after recovery, or the risk of relapse will be high.

If it looks like Strangles, you'll want the assistance of a competent equine veterinarian to make the decision about whether to give antibiotics and, if so, which to use. If his lymph nodes have abscessed, you can encourage them to break open and drain by holding warm, wet compresses over them several times a day, or you can have the vet lance and flush them. It's a mess either way, and the crud that contaminates the environment should be cleaned up and the area disinfected, or the

Strangles bugs can linger to infect the next horse.

If it looks like pneumonia, get a good vet on the case as soon as possible, because it's best to get the lab tests done (to identify the causing organism) and the appropriate antibiotic and other treatments started early in the game, before the lungs and pleura become damaged and riddled with scar tissue.

SPECIAL NOTE 14.3		SPECIAL NOTE 14.4	
ASPIRIN DOSE FOR FEVER ACCOMPANYING RESPIRATORY DISEASE		**BANAMINE™ DOSE FOR FEVER ACCOMPANYING RESPIRATORY DISEASE**	
800 lb horse:	3 grams	800 lb horse:	3 cc
900 lb horse:	4 grams	900 lb horse:	3-1/2 cc
1,000 lb horse:	4-1/2 grams	1,000 lb horse:	4 cc
1,100 lb horse:	5 grams	1,100 lb horse:	4 cc
1,200 lb horse:	5-1/2 grams	1,200 lb horse:	4-1/2 cc
1,300 lb horse:	6 grams	1,300 lb horse:	4-1/2 cc
1,400 lb horse:	6-1/2 grams	1,400 lb horse:	5 cc
To be given orally, once only.		To be given intramuscularly, once only.	

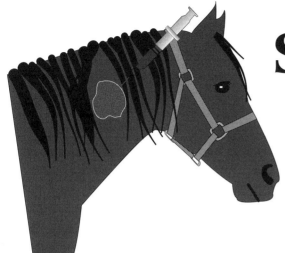

Severe Adverse Reactions to Medications

Every living creature reserves the right to react to a medication in an unexpected way, because every individual is different. As true as it may be that "a horse is a horse," each horse has his own unique arrangement of genes, his own history of exposure to allergens and irritants, and his own state of health. In fact, a medication that might behave in an "average" way in a particular horse on a particular day can result in a dramatic, unexpected response in the same horse on another day, under different circumstances.

Would you know what to do? Are you prepared? Or are you a gambler? If you give any medications to your horse, you have a responsibility to know that a dangerous adverse reaction can happen at any time, and you should be willing and able to deal with it.

What you see

Systemic anaphylaxis ("anna-fill-áxis")

This can be an immediately life-threatening condition, and the speed with which it appears and progresses will depend on whether the offending medication was given intravenously (which causes the fastest reactions), intramuscularly (slower), subcutaneously (slower still), or orally (the slowest). In many cases, the severity of the reaction follows a similar pattern: the intravenous dose brings the rapidly fatal reactions, and the odds of survival improve as the route of administration requires more time for the medication to be absorbed (with the oral route being the slowest).

In the very dramatic cases, within 30 minutes of receiving an intravenous injection the horse suddenly gasps or takes several "horrified" breaths, his ears might twitch three or four times in a bizarre, front-to-back fashion, he may suddenly become stiff and rigid as though gripped with terror, and then he collapses and dies.

In other cases, the reaction follows a more gradual course, sometimes not showing up for hours after the drug was given by the intramuscular, subcutaneous, or oral route. However, the outcome is often the same. A few hives appear on the skin, not necessarily near the injection site. The horse sweats profusely, with sweat literally drenching and running off his body. The hives quickly enlarge as more hives appear and spread, and sometimes they grow so profoundly that they actually coalesce into one or two huge lumpy plaques. Swelling may develop in the lower legs and under the belly. The usual noises coming from the abdomen may become loud and exaggerated, and the horse may pass diarrhea if he lives long enough. His muscles may twitch spastically, and he may lurch forward or kick back for no apparent reason, or he may break away and gallop as far as he can go, as though being pursued by some invisible monster. Meanwhile, he shows increasing respiratory distress, breathing heavily and with more and more wheezing, until he collapses.

Other cases might show only a portion of the above symptoms, and the severity of their reaction tends to be lessened when the offending medication was given in a more diluted form.

Survivors of systemic anaphylaxis often develop signs of severe colic, liver disease, or founder.

The allergic reaction

There are some technical differences between the anaphylactic reaction and the allergic reaction, but outwardly they appear the same: you see all or part of a sudden, unexpected, and often violent progression of alarm, anxiety, distress, hives, sweating, bizarre behavior, collapse and death. As with anaphylactic reactions, there is usually a delay of several minutes to hours between the administration of the medication and the onset of the symptoms.

The accidental reaction

By far the majority of so-called "reactions" to medications aren't allergic or anaphylactic at all — they're the result of an intramuscular medication accidentally being injected into a vein or artery, or an intravenous medication accidentally being injected into an artery. The main difference in the symptoms, which also helps to distinguish this event from an allergic or anaphylactic reaction, is how fast they appear: whereas the anaphylactic and allergic reactions usually occur after a delay of several minutes (and sometimes hours), the accidental reaction occurs instantly — BAM!!! — before the whole dose has even been injected. The horse literally falls away from the needle, flips over backward and convulses on the ground.

Mercifully, most of these cases survive, although a few suffer from residual brain damage (in some cases, no doubt, from head trauma), some are blind, and some have to be put to sleep because of injuries related to their fall.

What's going on inside?

In the case of the anaphylactic and allergic reactions, the cardiovascular system goes into shock, in which some of the blood vessels mysteriously clamp closed, others relax and pool the blood, and the heart loses its ability to pump efficiently, so it tries to make up for it by pumping faster. To make matters worse, the abnormally relaxed blood vessels allow plasma to leak into the tissues, causing swelling in, among other places, the membranes that line the respiratory tract. This makes it increasingly difficult to breathe, and in very severe cases, the animal literally suffocates.

In the case of the accidental injection of a medication into an artery, the reaction occurs because the drug goes straight to the brain, without any dilution or filtration by the liver, kidneys, lungs, or immune system.

Medications that were meant to be given intramuscularly are usually made of substances that won't dissolve in the blood, the most common examples being the white, creamy penicillin products, and the cloudy vaccines. When these medications are accidentally injected into a vein, the reaction can be a massive stroke — a clot that consists of a glob of the medication surrounded by cells from the horse's immune system becoming lodged in, and thereby plugging, a major blood vessel in the heart, lungs, or brain.

What would the vet do?

Ideally, the veterinarian would come prepared for anaphylactic or allergic reactions, carrying a pre-loaded syringe containing one of the only known treatments: *epinephrine*. That way, if he administers a medication and a reaction should occur while he's still on the premises, he/she can give the epinephrine on the spot, with no delays from having to run to the truck, rummage around, find the bottle, assemble needle and syringe, draw up the dose (let's see... how much am I supposed to give?), run back to the horse, and administer the medication. If the horse is going to respond to the epinephrine, it should be given immediately. Five minutes later might be too late.

Further care might include an emergency tracheostomy (so the horse can breathe), oxygen, intravenous fluids, intravenous steroid medications such as cortisone, and intravenous antihistamines. The epinephrine is often repeated at 15-minute intervals until the horse's treacherously low blood pressure comes back up to normal range.

As far as accidental reactions are concerned, there's really nothing that can be done after the fact because they happen so quickly — by the time anybody realizes what has happened, it's over. The horse should be examined and treated for injury, and life goes on.

There's no vet. What should you do?

Oddly enough, epinephrine is an over-the-counter drug. The kind you need is called "epinephrine 1:1000." The dose for an acute reaction of the non-accidental kind is 5-10 cc, intramuscularly (5 cc for a smallish horse, 10 cc for a draft horse, and frankly there isn't time to quibble about the in-betweens). If anything is going to save your horse, this is it, but be prepared for the worst.

If and only if you can get close enough without getting hurt, there are a couple of acupuncture points for treating shock that are worth stimulating. I've seen them work instant miracles, and I've seen them have no effect at all—you've got nothing to lose, so you might want to give it a try.

1. In your pocket, along with the syringe of epinephrine, you should also be carrying a brand new, unopened, 16-gauge disposable needle (no syringe—just the needle). Open it, and insert it at the edge of the gumline between the two upper front teeth (see diagram). If you've still got some safe working space, twirl the needle around a little and tap on the hub with your finger to stimulate the point.

2. Meanwhile, grasp the horse's upper lip (where a twitch is usually placed) and squeeze it as hard as you can. Use a twitch, if you have one handy. Pinch and waggle it around to stimulate the point that's deep in all that thick tissue.

In most cases, if either of these points is going to work, it'll work within a minute's time. There's no reason to continue beyond that timeframe.

If the horse recovers, move him to a quiet, darkened stall and keep him as comfortable as you can while you wait for the arrival of whatever veterinarian you can find. You'll want to be sure to watch for signs of founder. Don't, however, give ANY medications other than your one, emergency shot of epinephrine — you don't want to risk another reaction. A veterinarian can prepare for it, and you shouldn't have to deal with it once, let alone twice.

Do not give epinephrine if your horse is suffering from the immediate, falls-off-the-needle type of reaction associated with accidental intra-arterial injection.

STEP 1.
Give epinephrine

STEP 2.
Try a little acupuncture

AN ACUPUNCTURE "SHOCK POINT" ON A HORSE

It's located just on the gum-side of the edge of the gumline, between the two front upper teeth. Insert the needle, perpendicular to the gum's surface, to a depth of about 1/4 inch. Spin it back and forth between thumb and forefinger, and tap the hub a few times to stimulate the point.

STEP 3.
TLC and wait for the vet

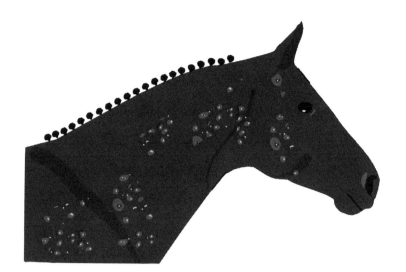

CHAPTER 16

Hives

(Urticaria)

An outbreak of hives on the shiny coat of a performance horse might seem like an emergency because of the effect it has on plans to show or compete, but in reality it's a potential emergency for another very good reason: it signals an ongoing hypersensitivity reaction, one that could escalate to full-blown allergic or anaphylactic shock (see *Chapter 15*).

Does this mean you should push the panic button every time your horse gets a case of so-called alfalfa bumps? Well, yes and no. Most cases of equine hives resolve as quickly as they appear, usually within 24 to 48 hours, and the cause is never figured out. But to shrug them off without a second thought is to invite disaster, because the horse is a practiced and infamous over-reactor to a variety of stimuli, and in most cases of fatal hypersensitivity, the groundwork for the reaction was laid months, maybe even years earlier. Which means that every outbreak of "the bumps" could be a dress rehearsal for the big one.

What you see

The onset is usually sudden — one minute his skin is clear, the next minute he's got a dozen or more bumps, and more are popping up every minute. The first bumps usually show up on the side of the neck, followed by the face, the chest, and the upper front legs. They may or may not be itchy. The bumps are initially distinct and steep-walled, and they retain a depression for several seconds when you press on them with your finger (this is called *pitting edema*). As they grow in size and number, they may coalesce into large plaques of swollen skin. If the outbreak also involves the tissues that line the respiratory and digestive tracts, there may also be respiratory distress (like a severe asthma attack, with wheezing and an increasingly anxious struggle to get air) and colic pain that leads to diarrhea.

Why is this dangerous?

The skin condition itself isn't dangerous. But it's only a symptom of an allergic reaction going on inside the body, and if that allergic reaction is widespread enough to involve the major organ systems such as respiratory and digestive tracts, and if it's escalating, the horse could be on a fast track to collapse and death.

The biggest mistake is complacency. Because the horse's body tends to be so overreactive, outbreaks of hives are seen pretty often, and as people become acclimated to the condition, they begin to see it as just a nuisance rather than a potential harbinger of disaster, and it gets "diagnosed" as "alfalfa bumps," spider bites, beestings, creosote allergy, and a number of other unsubstantiated "conditions" that satisfy people's need to pin a reason on things. As a result, the gravity of the situation is completely missed, and the chance to get help early in the process is completely passed by.

What would the vet do?

Because hives are the culmination of an allergic response that's been building for a long time, it's often difficult to figure out what the horse is reacting to — it's not, in other words, going to be some obvious "new" thing — it'll be something that has been part of the horse's environment for more than just a little while.

Figuring out the underlying cause is essential to resolving the allergy. The biggest culprit is medications. Lesser suspects include sensitivity to certain insect bites, food allergies, and inhaled dust/molds/spore allergies. The vet should take some time exploring the horse's history to try and identify a possible cause, then work with the horse's owner to formulate a plan of avoidance — stop all medication, or change to a different medication; change the stall bedding (some outwardly clean truckloads of sawdust are infested with biting mites, for example), cut down on the dust, etc.

Medical treatment is aimed at interrupting the allergic response, employing such agents as antihistamines and corticosteroids, but it should be remembered that this is only treating symptoms. Another thing to bear in mind is that corticosteroids can cause founder (see *Chapter 5*).

To truly resolve the problem, the underlying allergen must be identified and eliminated. To that effect, the vet has access to some diagnostic tests. Allergic skin testing is becoming more widely available to field veterinarians. Blood tests for levels of a specific antibody (allergen-specific immunoglobulin E) can search for hypersensitivity to some of the more common inhaled allergens such as pollens, barn dust, and molds. For chronic hives (hives that linger for more than a week), skin biopsies are often revealing.

There's no vet. What should you do?

STEP 1.
Assess the breathing

Don't panic — the vast majority of hives outbreaks in a horse are brief and limited to the skin. However, don't assume this is a "benign" case either. Stop whatever you're doing and assess the horse's breathing: Count the number of breaths per minute, and write it down (see *Chapter 19*). Look at his nostrils and chest wall when he breathes — is there any evidence that he's working harder than usual to get his air? Is he making any wheezing sounds when he breathes? Re-evaluate his breathing every five minutes to see if he's developing any respiratory distress.

STEP 2.
Assess the gut

Look for any signs of hypermotility in the gut: loose manure, belly pain, or exceptionally gurgly gut sounds (see *Chapter 19*). Re-check every five minutes for escalation of signs.

STEP 3a.
If it's a worst-case scenario, get help and stand by

If Steps 1 and 2 yield any worrisome findings, your horse might be in serious trouble, and his troubles could get out of hand in a matter of minutes. Get help.

Meanwhile, draw up a dose of epinephrine and stand by to give it in case the horse's condition worsens (see *Chapter 15* for information about the use of epinephrine). Do not give it if he seems stable or if he's improving — it's meant as an emergency treatment for a life-threatening, worsening situation only.

STEP 3b.
If it's just a pesky skin eruption, give no treatment

If, on the other hand, after 30 minutes you see no evidence that this particular hypersensitivity reaction involves any part of the horse's body other than the skin, focus your efforts on finding the cause rather than administering any treatment. Antihistamines, antiinflammatories, and corticosteroids are all prohibited in AHSA- and FEI-sanctioned events, and most cases of hives resolve within 24 to 48 hours on their own, so there's no logical reason to risk disqualification for a condition that really doesn't need treatment. Furthermore, any diagnostic tests your vet runs when you get home will be invalidated by these medications. Instead, just give him a cool bath and hold ice packs on his swollen eyelids to soothe and help calm his irritated tissues.

CHAPTER 17

The Well-Equipped Emergency Kit

F ollowing is a list of supplies that every performance horseperson should consider carrying on horse-accompanied travels. A great deal of thought went into selecting items that serve more than one purpose, take up a minimum of space, add a minimum of weight, and that can fit into a convenient carrying case such as a handyman's tool box, a duffel bag or a backpack. When two medications have similar actions, one was chosen and the other was omitted from the list — this not only helps to reduce the size and expense of the emergency kit, it also helps to eliminate confusion. When an over-the-counter medication can serve as well as a prescription drug, the OTC product is recommended. The prescription items included in this list are few and, without exception, they are familiar products that have been in use by veterinarians and lay horsepeople for many years. Nevertheless, their use is warranted only when backed by a prescription from your personal veterinarian and sanctioned by his/her advance expression of faith in your ability to act as his/her agent in an emergency where competent veterinary help is unavailable.

Some notes about special items on the list

The prescription items recommended in this book are specific agents that combat inflammation and pain (phenylbutazone and Banamine™), that alter the flow of blood (acepromazine), and that can protect a troubled eyeball without creating additional problems. Anitibiotics for systemic ("whole-body") use and mood-altering drugs (sedatives, tranquilizers) are *not* recommended, for reasons I'll detail in a moment. The goal of emergency care should be to stabilize your horse and make it safer to transport him to a competent equine veterinarian, not to "play doctor" and treat conditions to their conclusion without veterinary consultation. The best interest of the horse is, and always should be, the primary focus.

A word about antibiotics....

Giving antibiotics to *prevent* infection, rather than treat it, is based on flawed reasoning.

When an infection is already established, what you have is a huge crowd of identical bacteria that are all the same species, like a mass of clones, and the right antibiotic given at this stage can swiftly wipe them all out in one fell swoop and cure the infection.

But *before* an infection has become established, for example when an injury has just occurred and the injured tissues are *contaminated* with dirt and debris but not yet *infected*, what you have is a confused mess of many different kinds of bacteria, and each species is still trying to squeeze out the others by multiplying faster and getting established in the tissues first. It's a lively competition. If you give an antibiotic at this early, pre-infection stage, you won't prevent infection — all you'll do is influence which bacterial species wins the contest. Think about it: the contest winner is going to be the strongest bacteria that are *completely unaffected by your antibiotic!* You will have encouraged the growth of bacteria that are immune to your antibiotic by wiping out their competition for them, potentially creating a "super infection" that might be especially tough to treat.

Instead, the better course of action when you're dealing with a contaminated wound is to clean, clean, clean the wound and *physically* shoo as many of those bacteria out of the tissues as you can. If you succeed in cutting down on the sheer numbers of bacteria present in the wound, you'll increase the odds that the body's own defenses will be able to clean up the hangers-on. As an added bonus, the well-cleaned wound will heal faster than one that was left dirty and treated with antibiotics in an attempt to make up for the lousy cleaning job.

The cleaning should be done as soon as possible: It takes three to six hours after a superficial injury before bacteria contaminating the wound will have burrowed deeper into the tissues, where they can no longer be washed away.

There are quite a few antibiotics that are available over-the-counter, aside from the old standby penicillin: these include tetracycline, spectinomycin, and gentamicin. Don't waste your money on tetracycline — it can only be given IV, it's been known to cause severe adverse allergic-type reactions, and it can give a perfectly healthy horse a massive, fatal heart attack. Spectinomycin is pretty worthless in horses, and although gentamicin has a reputation for being a "strong" antibiotic, it has a relatively narrow spectrum of activity relative to the "bugs" that commonly infect horses. Besides, any antibiotics with names that end in -mycin or -micin can be ototoxic (cause deafness) and nephrotoxic (cause kidney damage).

Penicillin is also relatively narrow in its spectrum, and you've no doubt heard

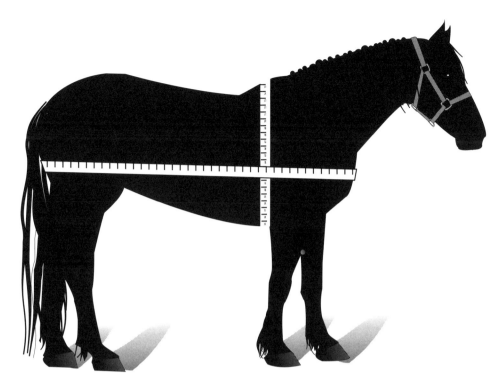

This 17-2 hand Friesian mare weighed 1605 lbs on a livestock scale. The state brand inspector estimated her weight at 1800 lbs. Estimating her weight with girth/body length yields a close "guess":

girth: 88 inches
body length: 68 inches
Formula: G^2 x BL÷330 =
88x88x68÷330 = 1596 lbs.

GETTING THE DOSE RIGHT

Horse owners and trainers traditionally overestimate the weight of their horses. When figuring doses of medication, an overestimated body weight can lead to dangerous overdoses. "Weight tapes," available at most feed stores, are often inaccurate when used on breeds of horses that differ physically from the "average" horse, the average being a generic equivalent of a Quarter Horse. Warmbloods, draft horses, Arabians, and the taller, leggier Thoroughbreds are likely to confound the weight tape because of their proportional variations from the "average horse."

Using a tailor's measuring tape and the following formula, the weight of your horse can be more closely estimated. If you're an "average person," you'll probably be surprised at how much heavier you thought your horse was.

When measuring the circumference of the girth, be sure the tape runs right behind the elbow and as straight up to the withers as possible. Don't stretch the tape, but try to get it to conform to the contours of the horse's body as closely as possible, and take your measurement when the horse has just finished exhaling.

The formula:
$[(\text{Girth})^2 \times \text{Body Length}] \div 330 = \text{Body Weight}$

about the dangers of penicillin-induced anaphylactic reactions — the more often your horse gets penicillin, the greater are the odds that he'll react to it. The "newer" trimethoprim-sulfa combination drugs have also been known to cause allergic reactions.

Another important reason you shouldn't use antibiotics in your horse is that, in most emergencies, whatever's causing his problem is highly unlikely to be bacterial. If antibiotics aren't going to help, and there are significant risks involved in their use, their availability over-the-counter is not reason enough to use them.

Antiinflammatories (inflammation fighters) and analgesics (pain killers)

These are essential to the well-equipped equine emergency kit. There are many drugs in this category available for horses, but some are only licensed for intravenous use (and unless you're a licensed veterinarian you should not be giving IV shots to your horse), some cause slowing of the intestinal motility (not a good idea in colic), and some cause drowsiness and dizziness (not a good idea from the standpoint of your own safety, and an unnecessary hazard to the horse if he's going to be trailered to a veterinary hospital). Therefore, only three products are recommended for your emergency kit: phenylbutazone ("bute") oral paste or gel, flunixin meglumine (Banamine™) injectable, and good old aspirin. Bute and Banamine™ require a prescription from your veterinarian.

Most tissue damage causes inflammation, whether that tissue damage is the result of an injury or an illness. In the case of injury, inflammation can expand the area of damage, often resulting in a wound that's twice its original size. In the case of illness, inflammation can set into motion a destructive cascade of events that perpetuates the illness, damages delicate internal tissues, and involves a wider range of body systems, making the illness more potentially dangerous. Bute and Banamine™ are good choices for the emergency kit because of their relative safety if given properly, their effectiveness against inflammation in many different kinds of tissues, and other beneficial effects specific to certain conditions that are discussed in the appropriate chapters.

As a painkiller, aspirin is only moderately effective in horses because it's so rapidly eliminated from the system — within two hours after giving aspirin to the horse, its pain-killing action is largely spent. But it's a potent antiinflammatory for certain conditions, it's a good choice for lowering a fever, and it's an invaluable tool in the treatment regimen for founder (for details, see *Chapter 5*). Best of all, it's a readily available, over-the-counter drug.

Sedatives and Tranquilizers

In an emergency situation, the administration of mood-altering drugs to your horse is strongly discouraged, and you will not find recommendations for their use in this book. It may seem that a sedative would make an injured horse safer to work on, but in many cases the converse is true — under sedation, most horses retain the ability to deliver a well-aimed kick, and all too often the aggressive reaction comes at an illogical time, when you least expect it and are least likely to be in a defensive position. Furthermore, the effects of these drugs on the horse are, at best, complicated and heavily dependent on a balanced status quo within the major organ systems. In the emergency situation, balance and status quo are woefully absent, and the use of sedatives and tranquilizers can cause dangerous, life-threatening reactions. And lastly, there are no drugs in this mood-altering class that leave intact the horse's ability to balance and navigate. Clearly, there are plenty of reasons not to use these drugs; there are no good reasons to use them. Leave this responsibility to someone who is certified, by his/her professional license, to understand the vagaries and intracacies of pharmacology and physiology under less-than-ideal circumstances.

Phenylbutazone ("bute") oral paste or gel

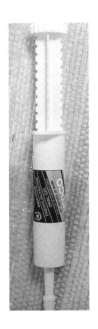

Benefits: Effective antiinflammatory and analgesic, easy to carry, safer oral administration, can also give some protection against the intestinal effects of endotoxemia in some cases.

Caution: Avoid personal contact (see comments below). High and/or prolonged doses are toxic to horses: can cause ulcers in mouth, on tongue, and in stomach and intestines, and can also cause kidney damage. Never give more than one dose in 24 hour period without seeking veterinary assistance for further instructions.

Obviously: Keep this and all other medications out of the reach of children in a locked medication box.

Warning: Use of this drug can disqualify your horse from competition.

Bute is available in oral (tablet, granules, paste, or gel) or injectable (intravenous only) forms. Use only the oral paste or gel. Do not buy the tablets to crush and mix with molasses because this will increase your own exposure to the drug — even though phenylbutazone is also sold in pharmacies for human use, the human population contains a small percentage of individuals who are sensitive to adverse effects from it, and those people should not be handling, mashing, mixing, and possibly inhaling the powder of the tablets. Even with the commercially prepared paste or gel, be very careful not to get it on yourself. Accordingly, keep this and all other medications out of the reach of children in a locked medicine box.

The most common use of bute is in the treatment of lameness and swelling from external injury. However, it may also have a role in the treatment of certain cases of colic. It is widely accepted that Banamine™ is the drug of choice in treating colic because in addition to relieving the belly pain, it also provides some protection against the cardiovascular effects of endotoxemia. However, research indicates that bute is more effective than Banamine™ in preventing endotoxins from slowing gut motility. For more on the use of bute in the emergency treatment of colic, see *Chapter 3.*

The oral syringes are marked, usually in increments of 0.2 gram. The dose recommended on some syringes is way too high for field use and for certain conditions. See the chapters on specific conditions for dose recommendations.

Flunixin meglumine (Banamine™)

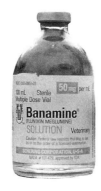

Benefits: Effective antiinflammatory and analgesic, relatively safe, injectable form can be given intramuscularly. Can also give some protection against the cardiovascular effects of endotoxemia.

Caution: Banamine™ is potentially toxic to horses, though generally less so than bute: prolonged and/or high-dose use can cause ulcers in mouth, on tongue, and in stomach and intestines, and can also cause kidney damage. Never give more than one dose in a 24 hour period without seeking veterinary assistance for further instructions.

Obviously: Keep this and all other medications out of the reach of children in a locked medication box.

Warning: Use of this drug can disqualify your horse from competition.

Banamine™ is available in oral (granules, paste) or injectable (intramuscular and intravenous) forms. If you can only carry one form, the injectable is more versatile because absorption of the oral form can't be guaranteed in cases where the horse's digestive tract is not functioning properly (such as colic and choke). If you can afford the expense and can carry more than one kind, the commercial paste is also useful for selected cases.

It is widely accepted that Banamine™ is the drug of choice in treating colic because in addition to relieving the belly pain, it also provides some protection against the cardiovascular effects of endotoxemia, and it does not slow gut motility the way many of the other antiinflammatories do. It is also used to treat lameness, pain, and swelling of tissues from injury or illness.

Aspirin

Benefits: Effective for fever reduction, short-term pain relief, anti-inflammation, and as an anticoagulant ("blood thinner"). Safer, oral administration. No prescription required.

Caution: Aspirin is potentially toxic to horses, though generally less so than bute or Banamine™: prolonged and/or high-dose use can cause ulcers in mouth, on tongue, and in stomach and intestines, and can also cause kidney damage. Never give more than one dose in a 24 hour period without seeking veterinary assistance for further instructions.

Obviously: Keep this and all other medications out of the reach of children in a locked medication box.

Warning: Use of this drug can disqualify your horse from competition.

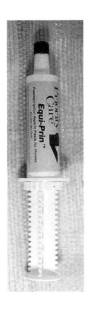

Aspirin has its limitations in equine treatment, but it also has its strong points, and there are some situations (treatment or prevention of founder, for example) where it's really unparalleled. It's cheap, it's safe, it's easy to give, and it requires no prescription.

Acepromazine

Benefits: Can prevent or reverse the abnormal, life-and-limb threatening constriction of blood vessels in the foot during founder, or in the muscles during myositis. Can be given intramuscularly.

Caution: When used in horses suffering from dehydration and electrolyte imbalances from overexertion, in whom the cardiovascular system is already weakened and in danger of collapse, the administration of *any* drugs, including acepromazine, can contribute to that collapse. Therefore, the administration of this and all other medications should be delayed until the horse has been treated for dehydration and electrolyte imbalance and has shown signs of recovery.

Obviously: Keep this and all other medications out of the reach of children in a locked medication box.

Warning: Use of this drug can disqualify your horse from competition.

Acepromazine is known as a tranquilizer, but it is not recommended that you attempt to tranquilize your horse in *any* emergency situation for reasons already discussed in this chapter. Rather, it is for the "side-effects" of acepromazine that it is included in this book — it has definite, powerful effects on the blood vessels in the body, causing abnormally constricted blood vessels in the feet and in the major muscles to relax and dilate. These effects have been well-documented, and the use of "ace" for these purposes, which has been published in many practical sources and has been shown repeatedly to be therapeutic when used properly, has become standard, accepted practice in the treatment of acute founder and myositis (tying-up syndrome).

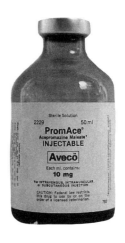

However, there are some dangers associated with the use of acepromazine in the treatment or prevention of myositis. If the horse is also suffering from heat exhaustion, he is more sensitive than usual to side-effects of any medications. Therefore, no medications should be administered to an overheated, dehydrated, electrolyte-imbalanced horse until his body temperature, fluid and electrolyte states have been addressed and he has recovered sufficiently to regain interest in his surroundings, show no further signs of abdominal discomfort, and voluntarily eat and drink.

The dose depends on the condition being treated — see the chapters on specific conditions for dose information.

Epinephrine 1:1000

Benefits: can reverse the abnormal, life-threatening constriction of blood vessels in the cardiovascular system during severe hypersensitivity reaction to a medication, also known as anaphylactic shock. Can be given intramuscularly. No prescription required.

Caution: Although this drug can save the life of a horse suffering an anaphylactic reaction, it would have no therapeutic effects and might, in fact, cause complications if given to a horse that is suffering, instead, from an accidental intra-arterial injection of a medication that was meant to go into a vein or muscle. See *Chapter 15*.

Obviously: Keep this and all other medications out of the reach of children in a locked medication box.

Warning: Use of this drug can disqualify your horse from competition.

The use of epinephrine in anaphylaxis is a last-ditch treatment to save a dramatically, violently dying horse, and it is by no means guaranteed to work — you should view the horse in anaphylactic shock as essentially doomed, and be pleasantly surprised if you manage to save him. For more, see *Chapter 15*.

The List

OTC= over the counter

RX= prescription required

Injectables

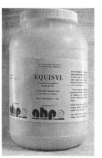

RX Banamine™

RX acepromazine

OTC epinephrine

OTC tetanus toxoid

OTC tetanus antitoxin

Orals

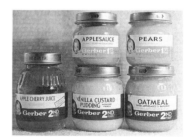

RX phenylbutazone paste or gel

OTC aspirin paste or gel (or tablets, to be crushed and mixed with suitable medium)

OTC electrolyte powder for endurance horses

OTC psyllium laxative

OTC mineral oil

OTC sweeteners, oral vehicles (molasses, baby food, apples, wheat bran, etc)

OTC probiotic paste or gel

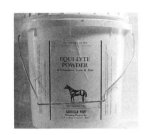

Topicals

RX atropine ophthalmic ointment 1%

RX "triple antibiotic" ophthalmic ointment (neomycin, polymixin, bacitracin)

RX proparacaine ophthalmic drops

RX Nexaband™ aerosol spray

OTC irrigating eye wash

OTC dimethylsulfoxide solution, medical grade

OTC povidone iodine solution

OTC "triple antibiotic" first aid salve

OTC nitrofurazone first aid salve

OTC hydrogen peroxide

OTC table salt

OTC Solvahex™ (for cleaning wounds)

OTC rubbing alcohol

OTC lubricating jelly

OTC epsom salts

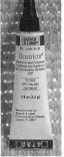
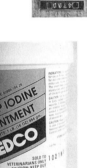
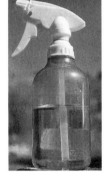

Miscellaneous

trigger-type spray bottle or 60-cc sterile, disposable syringe

measuring teaspoon

measuring cup

empty oral syringe from paste dewormer

steno pad and pencil

flashlight, spare bulb and batteries

douche bag

infant toothbrush

Tools and Instruments

stethoscope

18- or 19-gauge, 1-1/2", sterile, disposable needles (bring 10)

3 cc, sterile, disposable syringes (bring 5)

10 cc, sterile, disposable syringes (bring 5)

rectal thermometer

sharp hoof knife

whetstone or sharpening strop

hacksaw blade

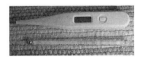
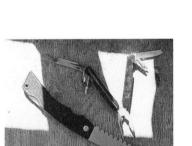

pocket knife

wire cutter

scissors

tweezers

screwdriver

hammer

pliers

clinch cutter (for pulling shoes)

Bandaging Supplies

tight-cell foam pad (backpackers' mattress)

rubber door stops (or other method of wedging up the heels)

gauze 4 x 4 sponges (a whole package)

cotton wool (bring one or two 1-lb rolls)

Type I bandage material (see *Chapter 18*)

Type II bandage material (see *Chapter 18*)

Type III bandage material (see *Chapter 18*)

Type IV bandage material (see *Chapter 18*)

single-leg splinting material (suggestion: a 3-foot length of 6" PVC pipe)

GelCast™ (bring 2 rolls) or Cool-Cast™

Ice packs (chemical cold packs, in case ice won't be available)

6" surgical stockinette, or leg from men's large longjohns

thick wound pad (suggestion: disposable diapers, Kotex™ thick sanitary pads)

The Science and Art of Bandaging

Much of your success in managing injuries will depend on your ability to bandage the injured area. Experienced trainers and performers take pride in their bandaging skill, but there's more to it than skill — you also must choose the right kind of bandaging material, which means that you must understand whether the horse's injury requires that you provide *compression*, *support*, or *immobilization*. In other words, do you want to squeeze the leg, or absorb some of its load, or make it rigid and unable to bend? Whenever you're in doubt about what a particular injury will require, you should assume that the injury is serious and apply a bandage that safely provides maximum protection. But to accomplish any or all of those three effects, you must understand what your bandage material is capable of doing. A bandage that is being asked to provide what it was not designed to provide will not only fail to help the horse — it might actually make his injury worse.

The Three Things a Bandage Can Provide

1. Compression, or pressure:

- to control bleeding
- to prevent or reduce swelling
- to hold damaged and displaced tissues in their original, pre-injury position
- to eliminate empty pockets ("dead space") where serum and debris might otherwise accumulate and interfere with healing
- to secure a medicated dressing and/or an ice pack over a wound

Other bandaging
materials you'll need:

PADDING:

a. cotton wool, 1-lb rolls, or

b. synthetic foam padding, or

c. pressed felt cast
   padding
   (sheet cotton is the least
   desirable padding for emergency bandages)

WOUND DRESSINGS:

a. non-stick pads (Telfa, or
   Release)

b. gauze 4 x 4 sponges

MISCELLANEOUS:

a. stretch gauze

b. duct tape

*A very stretchy material,
which can provide com-
pression but no support or
immobilization, can not
be made to provide sup-
port or immobilization by
simply applying it more
tightly — the higher ten-
sion will only increase its
compression.*

2. Load-sharing, or "support":

- to absorb externally some of the stress on internal load-bearing soft tissues
- to protect a limb from excessive load, such as when three uninjured legs are expected to carry the load of four because the fourth leg is injured

3. Immobilization:

- to restrict movement of an injured part and thereby prevent further damage, as when normal supportive soft structures, such as ligament, tendon, or muscle, have been mildly or moderately damaged
- to *completely* immobilize, as with a rigid cast or splint, when damage to internal supportive structures is catastrophic (such as in a fracture, or a severed tendon)

The Four Classes of Bandage Material

There are four classes of bandage material. Each class will provide its own unique proportion of compression, support, and immobilization, according to what *kind* of fabric it's made of, how *strong* that fabric is, *how* it stretches, and how *much* it stretches.

For example, a bandage made with a very light fabric that will tear under moderate tension will provide less compression and less muscle support than a bandage of stouter, heavier fabric that has similar stretch characteristics. A fabric that can stretch to twice its resting length (100% stretch) but which stretches in only one direction will provide less compression but more support than a fabric that stretches the same amount but in all directions. A bandage that has no elastic properties will provide better immobilization than a stretchy bandage, but if it's made of thin, lightweight material it will provide less immobilization and support than a stretchless bandage made of thick, heavy material. And a very stretchy material, which traditionally provides compression but no support or immobilization, can not be made to provide more support or immobilization by simply applying it more tightly — the effect of higher tension will only be an increase in compression.

If your stock of bandaging materials consists only of one kind of product, chosen because the colors are pretty or because it was on sale at the local tack store, you will be ill-equipped for the wide range of injuries your horse can fall victim to in his career as a performance animal and you'll be unlikely to help him when he needs your help most. For example:

- A horse with minor stocking-up in the legs might benefit most from a lightweight class I bandage that provides low-level compression, no support, and no immobilization — you certainly wouldn't want to "freeze" or immobilize that leg when exercise and movement are what he needs to eliminate the swelling.
- A horse with a leg abrasion might benefit most from a medium-weight class II bandage that provides medium-level compression, low-level muscle support, and no immobilization.

- A horse with a nasty laceration, perhaps with significant hemorrhage, might benefit most from a heavyweight Class III bandage that provides good compression, moderate muscle support, and minimal immobilization.

- A horse with a moderately damaged flexor tendon might benefit most from a modified class IV bandage that provides high-level compression, minimal immobilization, and, with the important addition of heel wedges, relief from tension on his damaged tendon .

- If the damage to the tendon is severe, adding splints to that class IV bandage will provide improved immobilization.

The Materials

To be adequately prepared to help your horse with bandages, you must have a variety of bandaging materials on hand so you'll be able to create at least one full-leg bandage of each class.

With very few exceptions, bandaging materials do not come with instructions and a description of what they can and can't do — it is assumed that the individual who purchases the bandaging materials has a prior, basic understanding of their capabilities and limitations. But the truth is, in many cases even the licensed veterinarian is unaware of the vagaries of each product. He/she may, through experience, choose the proper type of bandage material without knowing why.

Rules of thumb

- the more a bandage material can stretch, the less it can support and immobilize
- the less a bandage material can stretch, the better it can support and immobilize
- the less a bandage material can stretch, the greater is the danger that, when improperly applied, it will cause compressive/constrictive (tourniquet-like) damage
- applying a stretchy bandage with greater tension will not increase its ability to provide support or immobilization
- applying any bandage too loosely can permit it to shift and bunch, thereby increasing the risk of compressive/constrictive (tourniquet-like) damage

In other words, if you're faced with an injury that requires a pressure dressing in order to reduce or prevent swelling, but it's not essential to support or immobilize the leg, you'll want to use a very stretchy material for your dressing — one that puts a comfy squeeze on the soft tissues but that will "give" when the leg moves and bends, rather then tighten and compress.

If, on the other hand, you're faced with an injury that involves breakdown of important structures that normally support the leg, you'll want to apply a relatively rigid, non-stretchy bandage material that will restrict the leg's ability to move and

Many trainers believe that leg bandages must always be applied starting at cranial and progressing to caudal, and always rolling the materials so that they displace the tendon laterally (pull it to the outside). Research has debunked this belief — it really doesn't matter in which direction you roll the bandage. Furthermore, if you applied it tightly enough to displace the tendon, you'd risk damaging the skin and other soft structures.

For support bandages, spiral application absorbs more energy than figure-eights.

You can identify other examples of each class by testing the stretch. Take your ruler to the drug store!

bend, and in the process, you'll have to be even more careful than usual to protect against doing more damage by constricting the soft tissues (cutting off their blood supply).

A very common and unfortunate misconception is that a stretchy bandage can provide better support if you just put it on tighter. This is simply not true. All you accomplish by putting it on tighter is more compression and, therefore, an increased risk of constriction (tourniquet-like damage). Furthermore, the width of a bandage material does not affect its ability to provide support — contrary to popular belief, a roll of wider bandage material isn't going to provide better support than a narrower roll of the same material. And bandage materials with adhesive backing are not necessarily better able to provide support than bandage materials that aren't sticky. With these myths duly debunked, let's get down to learning about the various bandaging materials.

The Class I Bandage

Salient Properties:

This kind of bandage provides light compression, no appreciable support, and no immobilization. It is very stretchy: a 4" length of Class I bandage material can be stretched to a length of 10" (150% stretch) or more.

Examples of Class I Bandage Materials:

J&J Dynaflex, BD Tensor, 3M Vetrap, BD Elastic, Beiersdorf Cover-Roll Stretch, reusable Ace Bandage

Limitations:

Compression is minimal, support is nil.

Hazards:

Constriction damage will occur if applied at near-maximum stretch in a circumferential pattern (i.e., "girdling" the leg).

Proper Application:

In the emergency situation, a Class I bandage is most useful in holding a medicated dressing or ice pack over a wound. Because of its high stretch capability, the potential for bandage slippage is high, and if it slips, it's likely to bunch up and cause constrictive damage. Therefore, the bandage should be anchored in place to prevent slippage.

The Class II Bandage

Salient Properties:

This kind of bandage provides a moderate amount of compression for reducing or preventing vascular leakage, muscle hemorrhage, and/or swelling, and for holding damaged tissues in position and/or eliminating dead space. It is moderately stretchy: a 4" length of Class II bandage material can be stretched to a length of 8" (100% stretch). Because it has less elastic "give" than the Class I bandage, it can exert increased pressure (become tighter) when stretched by swelling or joint movement. It can be expected to provide medium support to superficial veins with mild support for muscles and tendons and mild restriction of joint motion.

Examples of Class II bandage material:

Bieirsdorf Lightplast, 3M Equisport, Kendall-Futuro Elastic, Sherwood Expandover, Champ Excel

Limitations:

Compression is moderate, support is negligible for injuries to major supporting structures of the leg.

Hazards:

Constriction of vascular and muscular structures with too-tight and/or circumferential application

Proper Application:

Useful for reducing or preventing swelling, controlling minor to moderate hemorrhage, and securing a dressing over a wound of mild to moderate severity.

The Class III Bandage

Salient Properties:

This kind of bandage provides moderate to high compression and can, if applied over bulky padding, provide moderate support and mild immobilization by limiting (but still permitting) joint movement. It is the least stretchy of the elastic-type bandages: a 4" length of Class III bandage material can be stretched to a length of 5" (25% stretch). Because it has less elastic "give" than the Class I or II bandage, it will exert the most pressure on blood vessels, muscles, tendons and ligaments when stretched by swelling or joint movement.

Examples of Class III bandage material:

Champ Support, Bike Conform, J&J Elastikon, Beiersdorf Isoband, Beiersdorf Elastoplast, Beiersdorf Comprilan, NDL Total Wrap

Limitations:

Support and immobilization are the best of the stretchy materials, but are still incomplete and will "give" under load.

Hazards:

Damage by constriction is a very real risk with Class III bandage material.

Proper Application:

The Class III bandage is effective for reducing or preventing moderate to severe swelling and moderate to severe hemorrhage due to injury.

The Class IV Bandage

Salient Properties:

Because it has no elastic "give," the amount of compression the Class IV bandage applies to underlying structures is a direct function of the amount of pressure used when applying the bandage and when swelling or joint movement occur in the bandaged leg. It should not be used as a compression bandage, because it will not release its pressure when the bandaged limb swells or when the joint of the bandaged limb moves. It should be used, rather, for adding some rigidity to a Class III bandage for partial immobilization of a joint, muscle/tendon, or ligament.

Examples of Class IV bandage:

Andover 150, Zonas adhesive tape

Limitations:

The Class IV bandage will not replace fully supportive, rigid devices such as a cast or splint — it is not meant to "treat" catastrophic injuries because it can not provide total support or immobilization. It is intended only to help prevent further damage that might occur after a catastrophic injury, before more appropriate treatment can be applied.

Hazards:

Risk of constriction and pressure/friction sores is highest with this sort of bandage and this material should, therefore, be applied over a padded bandage.

Proper Application:

The Class IV bandage is appropriate when partial immobilization and high-level support are needed to help protect an injured soft supportive structure such as muscle, tendon, or ligament. For significant immobilization, however, rigid splints should be added.

INSTRUCTIONS FOR SPECIFIC BANDAGES

Although the requirements for a particular injury will depend on a number of variables, there are some "cookbook" instructions for specific bandages that you should learn and be prepared to apply, with or without modifications to accommodate your horse's situation. Following are instructions for the four basic bandage classes, with specific instructions for altering them as needed when the injury is internal (muscle, tendon, ligament, bone) or external (cuts, punctures, abrasions, macerations). Elsewhere in this book, where specific injuries are discussed, you may be referred to this section for instructions on applying one of these bandages.

The Standard Class I Bandage

1. Treat surface wounds as directed elsewhere.

2. Apply the padding by unrolling around the leg evenly and smoothly, pressing out any wrinkles, ripples, or bunched areas with your fingers so there will be no sites of uneven pressure when the compression layer is applied. Conform the padding to the contours of the leg as well as possible without tension.

3. Just above the fetlock joint, apply a single revolution of stretch gauze to anchor the layer, applying just enough stretch to secure the cotton but not enough to apply pressure to the leg. Now figure-8 the stretch gauze over the fetlock and begin an upward spiral from 1/2" above the bottom of the cotton, all the way up to 1/2" below the top of the cotton, overlapping each revolution by 1/2 the width of the gauze, and evenly applying just enough tension to snug the cotton against the leg. Note: this is *not* a compression layer.

4. Choose a suitable Class I compression bandage material and apply it in the same pattern as the stretch gauze, exerting a 100% stretch (the Class I bandage can stretch to 150%). This should be tight enough to discourage slippage and bunching, but not tight enough to cause constrictive damage if applied smoothly, in a spiral instead of in a girdling pattern, and with even pressure. Extend this single spiral to the top of the cannon bone, leaving at least 1/2 inch of cotton wool exposed above the wrap.

5. With short, vertical motions, tear off the excess cotton sheet at both ends to leave a neat, 1/2 inch border of cotton sheet protruding.

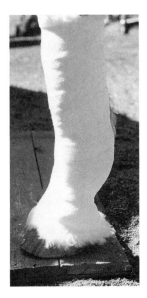 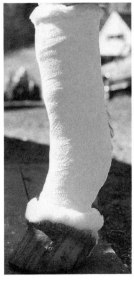

The padding layer is secured with stretch gauze under insignificant tension — the gauze merely holds the cotton in place.

The compression layer, in this case Vetrap™, is applied with even, submaximal tension.

The Standard Class II Bandage

1. Follow Steps 1–3 as for Standard Class I Bandage.

2. Apply a second padding layer and snug it down with maximum tension on the stretch gauze, following the same pattern [just above fetlock — down to bottom of bandage — up to top of bandage — back down with any remainder].

3. Choose a suitable Class II compression bandage material and apply it in the same pattern as the stretch gauze, exerting a 50% stretch (from 4" to 6" — because the Class II bandage is less stretchy, this is significant tension).

Because it is so well suited to face and eye bandages as well as standard Class II bandages, adhesive-backed Expandover™ is a good choice for the emergency kit.

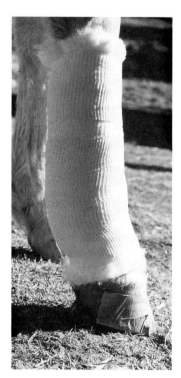

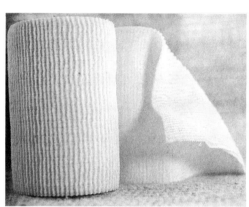

The Standard Class III Bandage

1. Apply a Standard Class II Bandage, all three steps as detailed.

2. Apply a third layer of padding directly over the Class II Bandage and snug it down with stretch gauze.

3. Choose a suitable Class III compression bandage material and apply it in the same pattern as the stretch gauze, exerting maximum stretch (from 4" to 5". This should never be done on a leg that has not been suitably padded first).

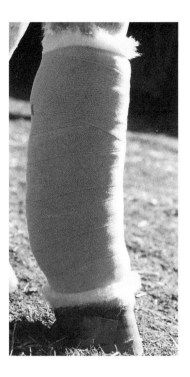

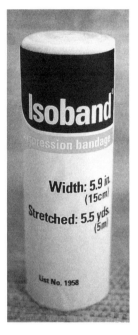

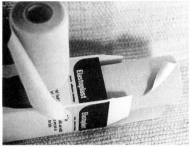

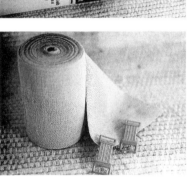

Elastikon™, Elastoplast™, Comprilan™ and Isoband™ are excellent Class III bandage materials for equine emergency use.

The Standard Class IV Bandage

1. Apply a Standard Class III Bandage.

2. Choose a suitable Class IV Bandage material and apply it directly over the Class III bandage, exerting as much tension as needed to compress the thick padding by at least 1/4" more.

For emergency equine use, standard 2" adhesive tape is the most universally useful Class IV bandage material. Others, including non-stretchy gauze (with or without latex treatment) are generally more limited in their use and would take up too much valuable space in the kit when compared with their usefulness.

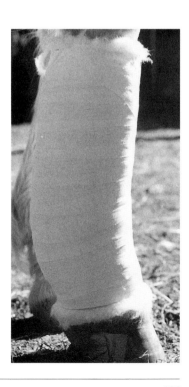

The Hemorrhage-Class Bandage

1. Apply one or more 1" stacks of 4 x 4 gauze sponges to the wound, enough to cover the entire extent. If the wound is too large for gauze sponges to be practical, use thick Kotex sanitary napkins or folded disposable diapers (absorbent surface against the wound). However, remember that the goal is to apply pressure, not to absorb — with this padding you want to create a focus of increased compression.

2. Secure the padding in place with stretch gauze, starting mid-wound and spiralling down, then back up, overlapping each revolution by 1/2 the width of the gauze. This is not a compression layer (the rest of the leg is not padded yet). Leave the bottom and top 1/2" of the padding exposed. Anchor the padding in place with a single revolution of a Class II or Class III adhesive-backed bandage material (suggestions: Elastikon™ or Expandover™) to keep it from shifting off the wound.

3. Apply a double layer of padding, preferably two revolutions of cotton wool, to protect the leg from damage by the compression layer, and secure with stretch gauze.

4. Choose a suitable compression bandage material and apply under near-maximum stretch, from 1/2" above the bottom of the padding layer to 1/2" below the top, but with maxiumum stretch applied to the "knob" of extra padding over the wound.

Under Class I or II tension and with a suitable water-soluble dressing under the stack of gauze pads, this bandage becomes appropriate for less dramatic lacerations and abrasions.

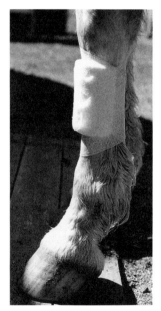
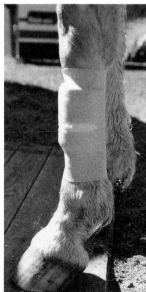
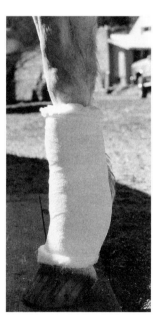

The Bowed Tendon Bandage

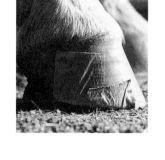

1. Thoroughly clean the bottom and outside wall of the hoof, then swab it with rubbing alcohol or acetone (oil-free nail polish remover) so tape will stick to it.

2. Prepare a heel wedge. [Suggestions: use a wedge of wood (see illustration), a 5" long roll of gauze, or 3 or 4 rubber door stops fastened together into a single wedge with duct tape.] Secure the wedge to the bottom of the hoof with duct tape as shown.

3. With the wedge in place, apply a Class IV Bandage.

4. To prevent the wedge loosening and shifting and/or to prevent the duct tape from wearing through, apply a hoof boot. If no boot is available, add sufficient duct tape, extending it up to the bandage.

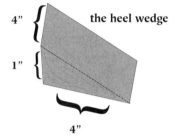

4" — the heel wedge
1"
4"

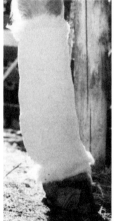

the Class I

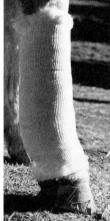

the Class II

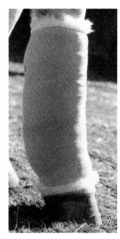

the Class III

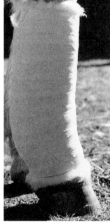

and the Class IV stages of the bowed tendon bandage

The Hock Bandage

Getting a bandage to stay over the hock, let alone getting it to stablize the hock, is one of the greatest bandaging challenges. The trick is to start by applying a separate bandage to the lower leg first, extending from pastern to the top of the cannon bone, then applying the upper leg component, overlapping the lower portion by 3". Start with a standard Class I bandage, and if the horse's needs indicate, layers can be added to both components (alternating lower first, then upper) until they're both the desired Class.

1. Apply a Class I bandage to the lower leg as directed.

2. Apply a single layer of cotton padding to the upper leg, overlapping the lower bandage by 3". Because of the awkward shape of the hock joint, it will be difficult to get this layer to conform to its contours. Concentrate on making the top part smooth at first, and then work small tucks into the lower portion so that the hock is evenly and smoothly covered. Secure with stretch gauze: start with a single revolution above the hock, then spiral down to 1/2" above the bottom of the upper-leg cotton layer, then spiral back up to 1/2" below the top of the cotton. Spiral back down with any remaining gauze.

3. Even if you intend to quit after a single layer, choose a Class II (rather than Class I) compression bandage layer that has adhesive backing — a non-adhesive material will be too prone to bunching around the hock joint, and a Class I material is likely to bunch and/or tear. When applying this layer, extend it about an inch *below*

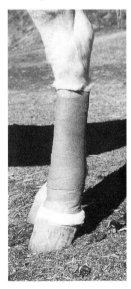

the "anchor" phase of the hock bandage

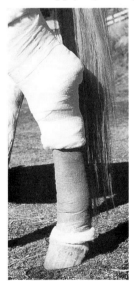

the padding layer applied

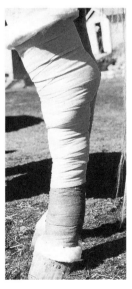

the single-layer hock bandage (additional layers can be added) *the bottom* of the cotton, onto the lower leg bandage, and, if desired, about 2" *above the top* of the cotton, anchoring the adhesive backing to the hair.

4. For additional compression, support, and restriction of movement, add successive layers, up to a Class IV, alternating and overlapping the upper and lower portions for added security.

The Hock Splint

To more fully immobilize the hind leg, apply the hock bandage as described, but extending the bottom of the lower component past the coronary band to midway down the hoof wall. Add alternate layers until the finished product is Class IV, then add splints:

1. Choose rigid materials that are strong but not too bulky, such as 1" x 1" wood, or broomsticks, or metal conduit. Cut two pieces: one to go on the inside of the leg and one to go on the outside, making their lengths appropriate to extend from ground level midway between the toe and the heel, along the leg, to at least 6" above the hock if you're planning to immobilize the hock joint, and just 2" above the hock if you're just planning to immobilize only the lower joints.

2. Place the splints on the inside and outside surfaces of the bandaged leg, the bottoms resting on the ground midway between toe and heel, and the tops centered on the inside surface and outside surface midway between front and back of the cannon bone portion of the leg. With a 2" wide piece of adhesive tape, create a connection between the two splints that will cross the front of the leg at mid-pastern, another that will cross the back of the leg just below the fetlock, another that will cross the back of the leg just above the fetlock, and another just above that which crosses the front of the leg, to prevent further damage to the tendon from bending of that joint.

3. To immobilize only the lower leg (not the hock joint), secure the splints in place with similar straps of Class IV material at the top of the cannon bone and across the front of the hoof wall, then add several more straps in between to hold the splints uncompromisingly in place. Then cover the whole thing, from bottom to top, with a standard spiral of the non-stretchy, Class IV tape, making it as tight as you can.

4. To immobilize the hock joint too, secure the splints as described above, but add similar straps of Class IV tape across the front of the leg above and below the hock, then angle a strap from above the hock in front to below the hock in back, and another from above the hock in back to below the hock in front. Finally, cover the whole thing, from bottom to top, with a standard spiral of the tape, making it as tight as you can.

The Knee Bandage

1. Apply a Class II Bandage to the lower leg, adding padding as needed to make the diameter of the bandage the same as the diameter of the knee joint.

2. If there is a wound on the knee, apply two revolutions of stretch gauze above the wound, then apply an appropriate wound dressing and anchor it to the gauze with tape. Figure-eight the dressing with stretch gauze, using just enough tension to conform the dressing to the wound.

3. Add two layers of padding, allowing it to rest on the lip of the lower leg bandage (rather than overlapping).

4. Choose and apply a suitable compression bandage layer.

5. For additional support and compression, add another layer of cotton over the entire leg, secure with gauze, and apply a final outer layer of Elastikon™ from hoof wall to unpadded skin of forearm — this prevents slippage.

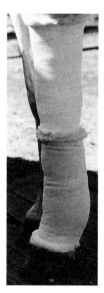 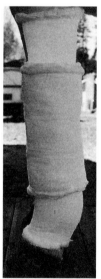 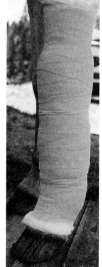

The thicker the padding in the central zone, and the greater the tension on the final compression layer, the greater the immobilization of the knee joint. An adhesive-backed compression bandage is preferred. Elastikon™ was used in this example.

The Head Wrap

To protect injured facial structures, sometimes a whole-head wrap is more effective and more likely to stay in place than a focal wound or eye dressing. Apply a focal dressing, anchored in place with adhesive tape, then apply the hood:

1. Apply a suitable stockinette over the head (suggestions: one leg from a Queen-size pair of pantyhose with the foot cut off, a leg from a men's large longjohns, or surgical stockinette material of suitable width for your horse's head size). Roll it up and slip over the muzzle, then unroll it up toward the poll, carefully cutting eyeholes and earholes as you go. Extend it only as far as necessary to encompass the ears in earholes (this will help anchor it). If necessary, make slits in the under-jaw section to enlarge the tube — don't let it "throttle" the horse.

2. If more compression or stability is needed, figure-eight an elastic-backed Class II or Class III bandage (Expandover™ works especially well), taking advantage of the natural "anchors" (the ears) and bridging the large lower jaw bones, rather than going behind them where the bandage might impinge on the throat.

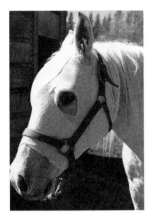 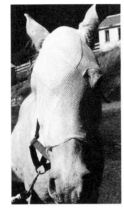

Expandover™ is especially suited for criss-crossing over the site of the wound because of its conformability and ease of application.

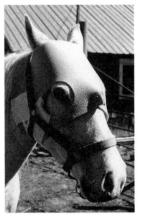

Makeshift Crash Helmet

When a commercial crash helmet is not available and protection is needed, a makeshift head protector can be fashioned from the close-cell, dense foam padding used for backpackers' mattresses. Make one in advance for each horse, as you'll not want to be snipping and fitting it during a head-bashing crisis. To apply, remove the halter and tape the rear portion behind the ears by running Expandover™ from the cheek section on one side, under the large lower jaw bones, to the other cheek. The front, face part should be folded back over the head, like a welder's helmet lifted up. Then bring the face part down and tape to the cheek pieces with Expandover™. If necessary, the bridge of the nose can be tightened by lifting up a "tuck" and taping with duct tape, as in the example pictured. The halter is applied over the helmet for additional security. The basic dimensions for making a helmet for your horse are given at right.

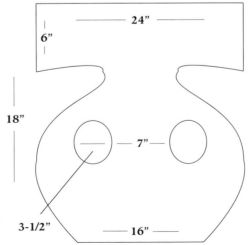

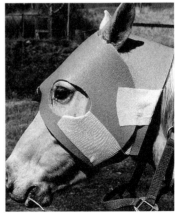

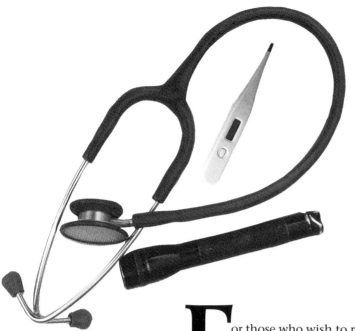

CHAPTER 19

Vital Signs

For those who wish to review the proper technique in assessing vital signs, the following pictorial series is presented. Interpretation of abnormal findings is covered in the appropriate chapters. For optimal performance during an emergency, all horse caretakers are encouraged to practice these techniques regularly — this not only hones observational skills, it also familiarizes the examiner with the normal values for each particular horse.

Pulse

Count beats/min by listening to the heart with a stethoscope (preferred method) or

by feeling the pulse in the artery that crosses the lower jaw bone (more difficult to do accurately, especially on a fidgety horse). To hear the heart, wear stethoscope so earpieces aim FORWARD, and "cram" the bell into the horse's left armpit.

Normal: 32-44 beats/min (adult)

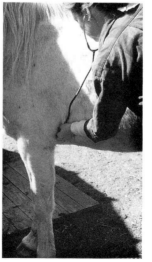
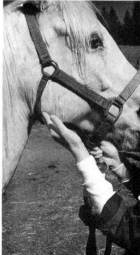

Rectal temperature

The electronic thermometer is faster (30 sec. vs. 2 min for standard mercury-type) and more accurate but more prone to error if the tip is not properly placed (if it's in an air bubble, for example). Lubricate the tip with lubricant jelly, insert 1" into rectum, and hold until ready to read. Holding the tail up sometimes annoys the horse — it's better to let it rest on the hand holding the thermometer.

Normal: 99-100.5ºF (adult)

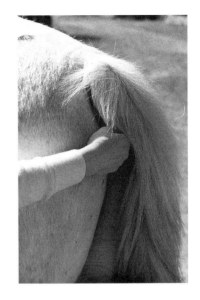

Gum color and CRT (capillary refill time)

Gently lift the upper lip and look at the color of the gums directly above the teeth. The normal color is light to medium pink.

To check CRT, blanch a spot on the gums by pressing with your finger. Release the

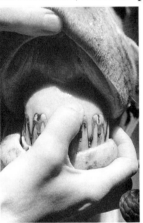
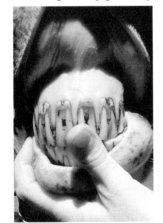

pressure and count how many seconds ("one thousand one, one thousand two,...") it takes for the spot to "re-pink."

Normal CRT: 1-3 sec.

Respiratory rate

Count the number of breaths/min by watching the nostrils flare, the chest move, or by listening to the throat with your stethoscope (preferred method).

Normal: 8-15 breaths/min

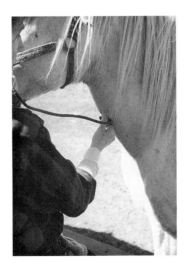

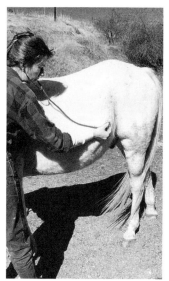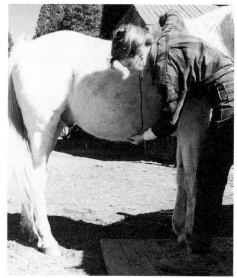

Gut sounds

Press the bell of your stethoscope (or your naked ear) against the abdomen in several sites on both sides and listen for gurgles, grumbles, roars, bouncing basketball pings, etc. Note how "busy" or "noisy" the gut is, or whether it's very quiet. Note also whether the sounds are short, abrupt, and staccato (not as good), or long and drawn out (better). In the location under the breast bone, listen for "sandpaper scraping" sounds, indicating sand colic.

Temperature of the extremities

Feel the ears and the lower legs for abnormal coolness. In the normal horse, these areas are cool or slightly warm, even when the weather is very cold. In advanced endotoxic shock, they're dead cold.

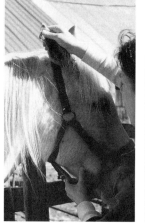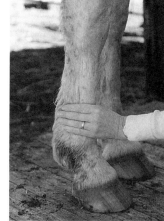

The skin pinch test for dehydration

Just above the junction of the neck with the shoulder, gently but firmly pinch a "tent" of skin. In the normal, well-hydrated horse, the skin will quickly spring back to its original position and the tent will disappear. In the dehydrated horse, the skin is less elastic and the tent lingers for a second or more. It's important that you pinch the described spot — just above a line drawn from the point of the withers to the point of the shoulder. It's also important that you practice this often in the normal horse so you have a frame of reference.

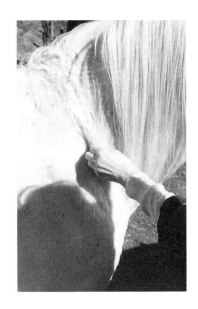

Check for founder

Feel the walls of the hooves, especially on the forelimbs, for excess heat. Even on hot days, the hooves are usually cool. If the horse is beginning to develop founder, they'll feel warm. If you're unsure, compare with a normal horse in the same environment. Also check for a digital pulse by lightly placing your fingertips over the back and side of the pastern bone below the fetlock. In the normal horse, the digital pulse is difficult to find. In the foundering horse, you can't miss it.

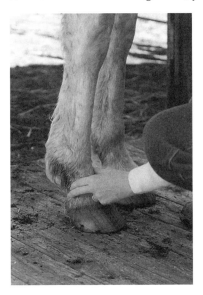

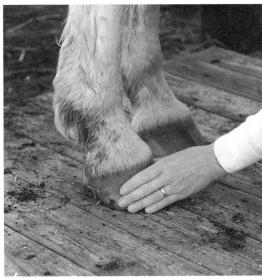

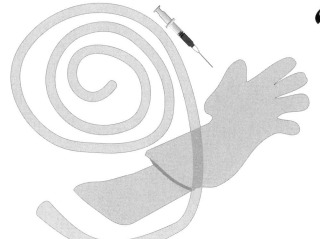

"I could have done that!"

Good veterinarians can make difficult procedures look simple. But I doubt if that's really the problem — there are just some people who, for reasons of their own, want to do everything themselves, and nobody has sat them down and explained the risks. There are three procedures commonly attempted by non-veterinary horse caretakers that are associated with unacceptable risk to horse, owner, and insurance company:

- nasogastric intubation ("tubing")
- intravenous injection
- rectal palpation

Following are some of the many reasons these procedures should be left for the veterinarian, even when a horse is in a crisis situation and the non-veterinary attendant truly believes his/her efforts can be life-saving. These caveats should convince even the staunchest do-it-yourselfer that it's just not worth the risk.

Nasogastric intubation

Properly passing a stomach tube requires

  1. carefully navigating a semi-rigid tube past lace-fragile scrolls of tissue in the nasal passages that will bleed like a stuck hog if even slightly disturbed,

  2. finessing the tube into the correct passageway when it reaches the fork in the road that leads to trachea (WRONG!) and esophagus (RIGHT!),

  3. advancing the tube down the esophagus without traumatizing its delicate tissues,

4. knowing how far is far enough to prevent backflow, and how far is too far so the stomach's walls won't be traumatized,

5. confirming that the tube is properly placed into the proper chamber before administering any medication,

6. removing the tube from the stomach without pulling a trail of medication up the esophagus where it might burn the walls, or up into the pharynx where it might get a second chance to go down "the wrong pipe,"

7. removing the tube from the nasal passages without injuring those afore-mentioned lace-fragile scrolls of tissue, and

8. managing all this without getting self or helper stepped on, struck, head-butted, etc.

There's a lot more to a botched tubing attempt than a bloody nose.

There's a lot more to botching a tubing attempt than creating a bad nosebleed, although that can be bad enough. Despite the fact that intubation is considered a "routine" procedure, potential mistakes are many, they're very easy to make, and the hazards of making any of those mistakes are virtually all life-threatening. They include

1. pneumonia, from accidentally depositing an oral medication into the lungs instead of the stomach;

2. damage to the esophagus from rough passage, rough removal, a rough-surfaced tube, or previous injury that left the esophageal walls more fragile than usual — damage to the esophagus can cause permanent narrowing, or stricture, that requires surgery to correct and is often irreversible;

3. a broken-off tube that requires surgery to retrieve — this is more common than most people know. The plastic that most stomach tubes are made of can become brittle with age (how long did it sit on the warehouse shelf before you bought it?), exposure to sunlight, exposure to temperature extremes, or just plain bad luck. Many a veterinary heart has sunken into rubber boots when the stomach tube is suddenly 14 inches shorter as it's being pulled out of the horse. The surgery is expensive, it's risky, and it's not the sort of responsibility you should accept without a great deal of thought.

Intravenous injections

A lot of non-veterinarians who are fond of giving intravenous injections to their horses seem to see an awful lot of "severe allergic reactions" in the horses they care for. What they describe, however, is *not* an allergic or anaphylactic reaction. Rather, it occurs when some yahoo, who fancies himself to be able to give intravenous shots without any special training, accidentally puts the needle into the carotid artery instead of the jugular vein. It's a *very* easy mistake to make — the carotid artery has

A CLASSIC CASE OF ACCIDENTAL REACTION

The stable manager, we'll call him Denny, was fond of giving Banamine™ intravenously to colicky horses at the breeding farm where I was the veterinarian on call. He'd seen how effective it was in relieving belly pain, how it completely resolved the vast majority of colics. He knew it could also be given intramuscularly, and that it worked just as well that way, but he seemed to like the drama of giving it IV (a show-off by nature?), and he merely grinned at my warnings that he was asking for trouble.

The trouble came much sooner than I expected, on a cold night in November. The patient was the farm's top stallion, whose pedigree and success in the show ring had earned him a stud fee of $10,000 and a long list of mares anxiously awaiting the coming breeding season. His colic pain seemed mild, and Denny was confident that he didn't need a vet's help. He drew up a full dose of Banamine™, pushed the needle into the horse's neck, drew back on the plunger to demonstrate that he was in "the" blood vessel, and started pushing the stuff in. BAM! Before he even got one-fifth of the dose administered, the stallion fell backward off the needle, flipped over onto his head and went into a violent seizure. Denny dashed to the phone and called me. "The horse is allergic to Banamine™," he croaked, his voice full of alarm. "It was an incredible reaction — I don't know if he's going to make it."

When I arrived, the horse had recovered from his seizure and was standing in the stall, shivering, a nasty bump on the back of his head, still cramping with colic pain. After a thorough examination, I pulled out my bottle of Banamine™, drew up a half dose and, while Denny's eyes got as wide as saucers, administered it — intravenously. The horse stood quietly. I turned to Denny and told him that what had happened was not an allergic reaction to Banamine™, but rather a reaction that any horse would have to any drug if that drug were injected into an artery. That's because an intra-arterial injection goes directly to the brain, rather than the gentler, more gradual route it takes when given intravenously (to the heart, through the lungs, back to the heart, then, in a much more diluted form, to the rest of the body). I think Denny got the message, but he never admitted it to me, and if he continued giving intravenous injections, he did so without my knowledge. I doubt if he has any idea how lucky he is that the stallion survived — not all do.

a nice, stout, muscular wall, unlike the jugular vein which has a paper-thin wall that is easily collapsed. And the carotid artery resides close *behind* the jugular vein in some regions of the neck and close *beside* it in other regions, so it's no trick to accidentally pass a needle all the way *through* the jugular vein into the carotid artery behind it, or completely miss the vein and penetrate the artery. Without a lot of experience, you'd have no idea you'd made this mistake until your horse flipped over and convulsed on the floor from an accidental intra-arterial injection. By then, obviously, it's too late. Why take the chance with IV medications, especially when there are so many effective treatment alternatives?

And there's one more thing about intravenous shots. Many of the injectable medications labelled "for intravenous use only" are caustic or otherwise irritating to the tissues if given by any other route — they'll "burn a hole" in muscles or subcutaneous tissues, so they have to be put into the vein where they can be buffered and diluted by the blood. Bute is a perfect example. Like other medications in this category, bute that accidentally gets injected outside the vein (like, for example, if the operator misses the vein, or pokes a hole through the vein, or pulls the needle out while there's still a drop of bute lingering on the tip) can cause serious inflammation in the tissues around the vein. Some of those tissues are vitally important, such as the esophagus, and the nerves that work the muscles of the larynx. The result can range from an ugly dimple where the tissues were burned, to permanent plugging of the jugular vein (which can cause swelling of the head and bulging of the eyes), to "roaring" from paralysis of the laryngeal muscles, to constriction of the esophagus (which can turn the horse into a chronic choker). Again, it's just not worth the risk.

Despite the fact that tubing is considered a routine procedure, there are a lot of mistakes that are easy to make, and they're almost all associated with potentially fatal results.

Rectal palpation

The walls of the horse's rectum are paper-thin. They can tear without warning, even if you're not being particularly rough. A rectal tear is almost always fatal. It takes years of practice before a practitioner has enough experience to be able to "feel" his/her way around the abdomen, and even with vast experience, a colic-case's findings on rectal palpation are often unremarkable, or confusing, or subject to interpretation. Statistics indicate that 50% of all colic cases fail to reveal any abnormalities on rectal palpation. This procedure is also one of the most dangerous from the operator's standpoint — it's a very effective way to get the tar kicked out of you. And, on top of all that, there's no way you'll ever convince a livestock insurance company that you were acting in the horse's best interest.

Bibliography

Allen Jr D, Clark ES, Moore JN, et al. Evaluation of equine digital Starling forces and hemodynamics during early laminitis. *American Journal of Veterinary Research* 51:122 (Dec 1990):1930-1934.

Allen Jr D. Pathophysiology and management of laminitis in the horse with colic. In: *Equine Acute Abdomen, Proceedings of the Veterinary Seminar at the University of Georgia*, 58-59, 1986.

Andrews FM. Acute Rhabdomyolysis. In: Veterinary Clinics of North America, Equine Practice 10:3 (Dec 1994): 567-574. Phila: W.B. Saunders.

Baird AN, True CK. Fragments of nasogastric tubes as esophageal foreign bodies in two horses. *Journal of the American Veterinary Medical Association* 194:8 (1989): 1068-1070.

Baxter GM. Management of proximal splint bone injuries in horses. In: *Proceedings of the 38th Annual AAEP Convention* (1992): 419-428.

Baxter GM. Acute laminitis. In: Veterinary Clinics of North America, Equine Practice 10:3 (Dec 1994): 627-642. Phila: W.B. Saunders.

Baxter GM. The steps in assessing a colicky horse. *Veterinary Medicine* Oct 1992: 1012-1018.

Becht JL. Analgesics for pain management in the horse with colic. In: *Equine Acute Abdomen, Proceedings of the Veterinary Seminar at the University of Georgia* 1986: 24-25.

Becht JL. Alterations in intestinal motility: effects on therapeutics in the horse. In: *Equine Acute Abdomen, Proceedings of the Veterinary Seminar at the University of Georgia* 1986: 26-27.

Beech J. Treating and preventing chronic intermittent rhabdomyolysis. *Veterinary Medicine* 89 (1994):458-461.

Belknap JK, Moore JN: Evaluation of heparin for prophylaxis of equine laminitis: 71 cases (1980-1986). *Journal of the American Veterinary Medical Association* 195:4 (1989): 505-507.

Bertone AL. Principles of wound healing. In: Veterinary Clinics of North America, Equine Practice 5:3 (1989): 449-464. Phila: W.B. Saunders.

Bertone JJ. Critical care in adult horses: restraint, analgesia and antiinflammatory support. *Veterinary Medicine* 88(1993):10661085.

Black JB. Hindlimb lameness of the western working stock horse. In: *Proceedings of the 37th Annual Convention Proceedings of the AAEP*, 1991: 393-404.

Booth L. Early wound management in the horse. *Equine Practice* 14:7 (July/Aug 1992): 24-33.

Boyd JS. Selection of sites for intramuscular injections in the horse. *Veterinary Record* 121:9 (1987): 197-200.

Buechner-Maxwell V. Airway hyperresponsiveness. *Compendium on Continuing Education* 15 (1993):1379-1383.

Cambridge H, Lees P, Hooke RE et al. Antithrombotic actions of aspirin in the horse. *Equine Veterinary Journal* 23:2 (Mar 1991): 123-127.

Carthy RN, Hutchins DR. Survival rates and post-operative complications after equine colic surgery. *Australian Veterinary Journal* 65 (1988):40-43.

Chaffin MK and Carter GK. Equine bacterial pleuropneumonia. Part I. Epidemiology, pathophysiology and bacterial isolates. *Compendium on Continuing Education* 15 (1993):1642-1649.

Cohen ND, Roussel AJ, Lumsden JH et al. Alterations of fluid and electrolyte balance in Thoroughbred racehorses following strenuous exercise during training. *Canadian Journal of Veterinary Research* 57 (1993):9-13.

Dabareiner RM, White II NA. Large colon impaction: retrospective study in 147 horses. In: *Proceedings of the 40th Annual AAEP Convention* (1994):121-122.

Dalgliesh R, Love S, Pirie HM, et al. An outbreak of strangles in young ponies. *Veterinary Record* 132 (1993):528-531.

Doran R. Field management of simple intestinal obstruction in horses. *Compendium on Continuing Education* 15:3 (Mar 1993): 463-471.

Dotson SJ. Desmitis of the accessory ligament of the deep digital flexor tendon: 27 cases (1986-1990). *Equine Veterinary Journal* 23 (1991):438-444.

Douglas Byars T, Becht JL. Pleuropneumonia. In: Veterinary Clinics of North America, Equine Practice 7:1 (1991): 63-78. Phila: W.B. Saunders.

Ecker GL and Lindinger MI. Fluid and electrolytes: in short supply? Part 1. *Equine Athlete* 7:3(1994):15-17.

Evans AG. Southborough, MA. Urticaria in horses. *Compendium on Continuing Education* 15 (1993):622-632.

Evans AG. Urticaria in horses. *Compendium on Continuing Education* 15:4 (April 1993): 626-631.

Fessler JF. Hoof injuries. In: Veterinary Clinics of North America, Equine Practice 5:3 (1989): 643-664. Phila: W.B. Saunders.

Fischer D, Easley J. Proper restraint. *Large Animal Veterinarian* Nov/Dec 1993: 14-33.

Frazier DL. Synchronous diaphragmatic flutter. In: *Proceedings of the 37th Annual Convention of the AAEP* (1991): 833-834.

Freeman DE, Ferrante PL, Chalupa W, et al. Effects of dioctyle sodium sulfasuccinate and magnesium sulfate on fecal composition and output in normal horses. In: *Proceedings of the 37th Annual Convention of the AAEP* (1991): 663-5664.

French DA. Soft tissue emergency in adult horses. In: Veterinary Clinics of North America, Equine Practice 10:3 (Dec 1994): 575-590. Phila: W.B. Saunders.

Geiser DR, Andrews FM, Sommardahl CS. Electrolyte and fluid changes in the event horse. In: *Proceedings of the 39th Annual AAEP Convention* (1993) : 189-190.

Genovese RL. Prognosis of superficial flexor tendon and suspensory ligament injuries. In: *Proceedings of the 39th Annual AAEP Convention* (1993): 17-20.

Goetz TE. Anatomic, hoof, and shoeing considerations for the treatment of laminitis in horses. *Journal of the American Veterinary Medical Association* 190:10 (1987): 1323-1332.

Green S. Equine tetanus: a review of the clinical features and current perspectives on treatment and prophylaxis. In: *Proceedings of the 38th Annual AAEP Convention* (1992): 299-306.

Green EM, Garner HE, Sprouse RF. Laminitis/endotoxemia: pathophysiology and therapeutic strategy. *Proceedings of ACVIM* 6(1988):323-328.

Green E, Allen K, Becht J, et al. Endotoxemia (roundtable discussion). *Equine Practice* 15:2 (Feb 1993): 2-13.

Hardy J, Stewart RH, Beard WL, et al. Complications of nasogastric intubation in horses: nine cases (1987-1989). *Journal of the American Veterinary Medical Association* 201(1992):483-486.

Harris P: Equine rhabdomyolysis syndrome. *In Practice*, Vol 11 (1989): 3-8.

Henderson A. Equine acupuncture. *Large Animal Veterinarian* Sept/Oct 1990: 7-9.

Hormanski CE. Management of anaphylactic reactions in the horse. In: *Proceedings of the 37th Annual Convention of the AAEP* (1991): 61-70.

Howard RD, Stashak TS, Baxter GM. Evaluation of occlusive dressings for management of full-thickness excisional wounds on the distal portion of the limbs of horses. *American Journal of Veterinary Research* 54:2 (1993):150-154.

Hunt RJ, Allen D, Moore JN. Effect of endotoxin administration on equine digital hemodynamics and starling forces. *American Journal of Veterinary Research* 51:11(Nov 1990): 1703-1707.

Hyde J. Management of some common equine problems. *Veterinary Surgeon* 151993):9-12.

Keegan KG, Baker GJ, Boero MJ, et al. Measurement of suspensory ligament strain using a liquid mercury strain gauge: evaluation of strain reduction by support bandaging and alteration of hoof wall angle. In: *Proceedings of the 37th Annual Convention of the AAEP* (1991): 243-244.

Kristula M, McDonnell S. Effect of drinking water temperature on consumption and preference of water during cold weather in ponies. In: *Proceedings of the 40th Annual AAEP Convention* (1994): 95-98.

Lakritz J, Wilson WE, Berry CR, Schrenzel MD et al. Bronchointerstitial pneumonia and respiratory distress in young horses: clinical, clinicopathologic, radiographic and pathological findings in 23 cases (1984-1989). *Journal of Veterinary Internal Medicine* 7 (1993):277-288.

Lengel J. AHSA amends medication rule. *Equine Practice* 11:9(Oct 1989): 9-10.

Lengel, JG. Understanding the 1993 AHSA Drugs and Medications Rule (a pamphlet), March 1, 1993. American Horse Shows Association, Inc. 220 East 42nd Street, Fourth Floor, New York, NY 10017-5806. 212-972-2472; The AHSA Drugs and Medications Program, 3780 Ridge Mill Drive, Hilliard, OH 43026, 800-MED-AHSA.

Lindsay WA. Equine bandaging techniques. In: Veterinary Clinics of North America, Equine Practice 5:3 (1989): 513-538. Phila: W. B. Saunders.

Lindsay WA. Repairing facial wounds in horses. *Veterinary Medicine* July 1989: 709-718.

MacAllister CG, Morgan SJ, Borne AT et al. Comparison of adverse effects of phenylbutazone, flunixin meglumine and ketoprofen in horses. *Journal of the American Veterinary Medical Association* 202 (1993):71-77.

Mair TS, deWesterlaken LV, Cripps PJ et al. Diarrhea in adult horses: a survey of clinical cases and an assessment of some prognostic indices. *Veterinary Record* 126 (1990): 479-481.

McDiarmid AM. Eighteen cases of desmitis of the accessory ligament of the deep digital flexor tendon. *Equine Veterinary Education* 6(1994):49-56.

Meschter CL, Gilbert M, Ktook L, et al. The effects of phenylbutazone on the intestinal mucosa of the horse: a morphological, ultrastructural, and biochemical study. *Equine Veterinary Journal* 22:4 (Jul 1990): 255-263.

Miller RM. Submissive behavior associated with flight deprivation in the horse. In: *Proceedings of the 37th Annual Convention of the AAEP* (1991): 405-408.

Millichamp NJ. Ocular Trauma. In: Veterinary Clinics of North America, *Equine Practice* 8:3 (1993): 521-536. Phila: W. B. Saunders.

Modransky P, Welker B, Pickett JP. Management of facial injuries. In: Veterinary Clinics of North America, Equine Practice 5:3 (1989): 665-682. Phila: W. B. Saunders.

Mohammed JO, Lowe J, Strug Jr JJ. Phenylbutazone and flunixin meglumine: establishing maximum allowable levels for American Horse Shows Association rules. In: *Proceedings of the 37th Annual Convention of the AAEP* (1991): 47-60.

Moore CP. Eyelid and Nasolacrimal Disease. In: Veterinary Clinics of North America, Equine Practice 8:3 (1992): 499-520. Phila: W. B. Saunders.

Moore JN. Pathophysiology of intestinal ischemia and endotoxemia. *Equine Practice* 14:9 (Oct 1992): 13-21.

Moore JN. The decision for surgery. In: Equine Acute Abdomen, *Proceedings of the Veterinary Seminar at the University of Georgia* (1986): 33-34.

Morris DD. Antiendotoxin serum: therapeutic rationale and clinical perspectives. *Compendium on Continuing Education*, 11:9 (Sept 1989): 1096.

Moyer W. Factors affecting the prognosis of limb injuries. *Compendium on Continuing Education* 10:4 (1988): 499-504.

Moyer W, Fisher JRS. Bucked shins: effects of differing track surfaces and proposed training regimens. In: *Proceedings of the 37th Annual Convention of the AAEP* (1991): 541-548.

Moyer W, Redden RR. Therapy for chronic severe laminitis—recurrence is common in severely affected horses. *Equine Veterinary Journal* 21(1989): 317-318.

Mueller POE, Parks AH, Baxter GM. Small intestinal diseases of horses: diagnosis and surgical intervention. *Veterinary Medicine* (Oct 1992): 1030-1036.

Murray MJ. Diarrhea in adult horses. *Journal of Equine Veterinary Science* 13 (1993):374-376.

Nasisse MP, Nelms S. Equine Ulcerative Keratitis. In: Veterinary Clinics of North America, Equine Practice 8:3, 537-556, 1992. Phila: W. B. Saunders.

Nielson IL, Jacobs KA, Huntington PJ et al. Adverse reaction to procaine penicillin G in horses. *Australian Veterinary Journal* 65:6 (1988): 181-184.

Peloso JG, Watkins JP, Keele SR, et al. Bilateral stress fractures of the tibia in a racing American Quarter Horse. *Journal of the American Veterinary Medical Association* 203:6(Sept 1993): 801-805.

Petrites-Murphy M. Anaphylactic reactions: rare, but sometimes lethal. *Equine Disease Quarterly* 2(3):5-6, 1994.

Pool RR. Pathophysiology of athletic injuries of the horse: bones, joints and tendons. *Association of Equine Sports Medicine Quarterly* 3:2(1988):, 23-29.

Powell DG. Viral respiratory disease of the horse. In: Veterinary Clinics of North America, Equine Practice 7:1(1991): 27-52. Phila: W. B. Saunders.

Prasse KW, Allen Jr. D, Moore JN, et al. Evaluation of coagulation and fibrinolysis during the prodromal stages of carbohydrate-induced acute laminitis in horses. *American Journal of Veterinary Research* 51:12(Dec 1990): 1950-1955.

Racklyeft DJ, Love DN. Influence of head posture on the respiratory tract of healthy horses. *Australian Veterinary Journal* 67:11(Nov 1990): 402-405.

Rebhun WC. Ocular emergencies. In: Veterinary Clinics of North America, Equine Practice 10:3 (Dec 1994): 591-602. Phila: W. B. Saunders.

Redden RF. 18° elevation of the heel as an aid to treating acute and chronic laminitis in the equine. In: *Proceedings of the 38th Annual AAEP Convention* (1992): 375-380.

Reed SM. Management of head trauma in horses. *Compendium on Continuing Education* 15(1993):270-273.

Ridgway KJ. Exertional myopathies. In: *Proceedings of the 37th Annual Convention of the AAEP* (1991): 839-844.

Schlipf Jr JW, Baxter GM. Nonsurgical conditions of the equine gastrointestinal tract. *Veterinary Medicine* Oct 1992: 1019-1025.

Schoster JV: Surgical repair of equine eyelid lacerations. *Veterinary Medicine* 83:10(1988): 1042-1049.

Schwink KL. Equine Uveitis. In: Veterinary Clinics of North America, Equine Practice 8:3(1992): 557-574. Phila: W. B. Saunders.

Semrad SD, Douglas Byars T. Pleuropneumonia and pleural effusion: diagnosis and treatment. *Veterinary Medicine* June 1989: 627-635.

Smith HL, Chalmers GA, Wedel R. Acute hepatic failure (Theiler's disease) in a horse. *Canadian Veterinary Journal* 32:6(Jun 1991): 362-364.

Spurlock SL and Hanie EA. Antibiotics in the treatment of wounds. In: Veterinary Clinics of North America, Equine Practice 5:3(1989): 465-482. Phila: W. B. Saunders.

Sweeney CR, Holcombe SJ, Barningham SC, et al. Aerobic and anaerobic bacterial isolates from horses with pneumonia or pleuropneumonia and antimicrobial susceptibility patterns of the aerobes. *Journal of the American Veterinary Medical Association* 198:5(Mar 1991): 839-842.

Tomlinson CM. Exhausted horse syndrome. In: *Proceedings of the 37th Annual Convention of the AAEP* (1991): 835-838.

Traub-Dargatz JL. Bacterial pneumonia. In: Veterinary Clinics of North America, Equine Practice 7:1(1991): 53-62. Phila: W. B. Saunders.

Traub-Dargatz JL, Salman MD, Voss JL. Medical problems of adult horses, as ranked by equine practitioners. *Journal of the American Veterinary Medical Association* 198:10 (May 1991): 745-1747.

Trent AM, Cox V. Pressure wraps: a comparison of surface pressure peaks and durations. In: *Proceedings of the 37th Annual Convention of the AAEP* (1991): 245-246.

Trotter GW. Principles of early wound management. In: Veterinary Clinics of North America, Equine Practice 5:3(1989): 483-498. Phila: W. B. Saunders.

Trout DR, Hornof WJ, Linford RL et al. Scintigraphic evaluation of digital circulation during the developmental and acute phases of equine laminitis. *Equine Veterinary Journal* 22:6 (Nov 1990): 416-421.

Underdal RG, Park BJ, Yates CS. A comparative report on the support characteristics of bandaging products. (unpublished paper). C. Steven Yates, Head Athletic Trainer, Bowman Gray School of Medicine, Wake Forest University, Post Office Box 7329, Winston-Salem, NC, 27109, 910-759-5955.

Urquhart K. Nasogastric intubation of the horse. *In Practice*, May (1987):84-85.

Whitley RD, Miller TR, Wilson JH. Therapeutic considerations for equine recurrent uveitis. *Equine Practice* 15(1993):16-23.

White II NA. Intestinal function and dysfunction in the horse. In: *Equine Acute Abdomen, Proceedings of the Veterinary Seminar at the University of Georgia* (1986): 5-11.

White II JA. Risk and prognosis of the equine patient with colic. In: *Equine Acute Abdomen, Proceedings of the Veterinary Seminar at the University of Georgia* (1986): 50-51.

Whitehair KJ, Cox JH, Coyne CP et al. Esophageal obstruction in horses. *Compendium on Continuing Education* 11:1 (Jan 1990): 91.

Whitley RD, Miller TR. Therapeutic considerations for equine recurrent uveitis. *Equine Practice* 15:5 (May 1993): 16-23.

Wilson, James F., DVM, JD. Law and Ethics of the Veterinary Profession. 1988. Yardley, PA Priority Press Ltd.

Zamos DT. Effects of three immobilization techniques on strain of superficial and deep digital flexor tendon in equine cadaver limbs. In: *Proceedings of the 20th Annual Conference of the Veterinary Orthopedic Society* (1993): 1.

Index

tibial stress fracture
  common causes of 86
  emergency treatment of 87
  ideal treatment of, by veterinarian 86-87
  internal events in 86
  veterinary follow up in the treatment of 87
toes, resentment of pressure on, and founder 43
tongue, injury to 114
tools and instruments, for emergency kit (list) 179-180
tooth, dislodged 114, 115
trailering, risk factor for respiratory disease 157
training, its role in bucked shins and shin splints 78, 80
tranquilizers 175
tube, stomach, the hazards of attempting to pass 200-201
turpentine, as colic remedy, as founder remedy 1
tying-up (see myositis)

United States Department of Agriculture (USDA), and drugs 3
uveitis
  recurrent (see moon blindness)
  symptoms and signs 138

virus, as cause of respiratory disease 158
vital signs
  how to check 196-199
  in colic 29

wedge, heel
  in the treatment of bowed tendon 74-75, 191
  in the treatment of founder 47, 50, 51, 191
wounds
  facial (see head wounds)
  head (see head wounds)